Uniquely, Fully, Enough

Uniquely, Fully, Enough

The Neurodivergent Parenting Journey

A Memoir and Handbook

Vicki Christensen

Empowered Voice Press

ISBN (Paperback): 979-8-9941972-0-2
ISBN (eBook): 979-8-9941972-1-9

Book design by the Aaxel Author Group
www.aaxelauthorgroup.com

Cover artwork by Vincent-louis Apruzzese

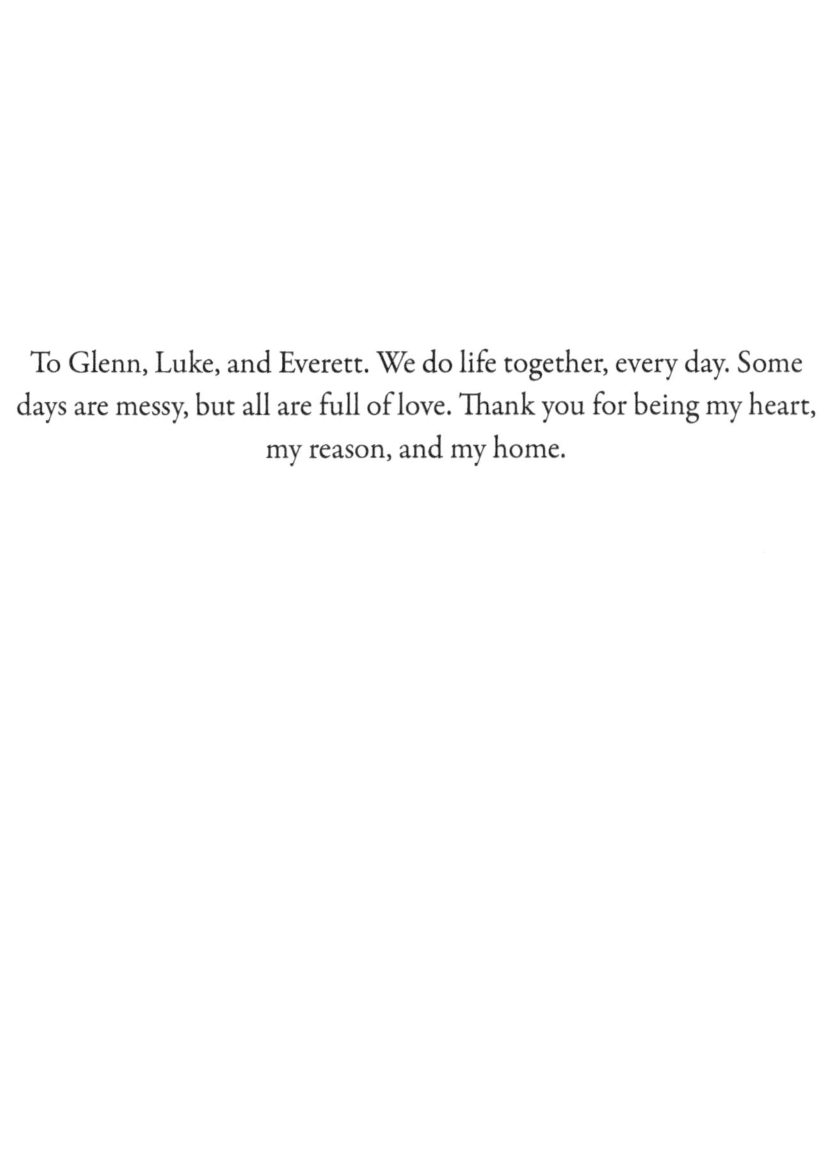

To Glenn, Luke, and Everett. We do life together, every day. Some days are messy, but all are full of love. Thank you for being my heart, my reason, and my home.

CONTENTS

Introduction

I should start by saying that I never aspired to write a book. Honestly, for the past 21 years, I've been a tired mom who loves her family and keeps stumbling forward one day at a time. My oldest son, Luke, has a rare chromosome disorder, and raising him—my wonderfully neurodivergent son—and his brother has been the greatest, hardest, and most meaningful journey of my life. Along the way, and by necessity, I became a special education advocate. For the past 15 years, I've been sitting at IEP tables, learning the system, and helping not only Luke but also other parents find their footing.

This book is part memoir, part handbook. Each chapter starts with a story and ends with a *Love Lesson from a Mom.*

It's me sharing our life and being real about the ups and downs of parenting a neurodivergent child. It's equal parts messy, raw, with a touch of humor—because sometimes if we don't laugh, we'll cry. I've included a *Handbook Highlights* section at the end, which organizes the practical takeaways from each chapter into bullet points. This allows readers to quickly reference specific guidance when they don't have the bandwidth to read a whole story but desperately need a tip.

This was the book I needed in my early years as a parent but couldn't find. A book that was real and relatable, that didn't sugarcoat the hard parts or speak in clinical terms but instead was available when I felt scared, overwhelmed and alone. I wanted a book that would make me laugh when the moments were absurd, cry when the truth hit hard and remind me that I wasn't the only parent navigating a path that looked nothing like the one I once imagined. This book is my way of offering that to others and my intent is that it becomes a source of comfort and empowerment for anyone traveling a similar road.

Most of what I've learned has come through trial, error, and doing a lot of things "wrong" the first time around. Parenting a neurodivergent child isn't about getting it perfect. It's about showing up, staying present, and finding joy in unexpected places.

Take what helps and leave what doesn't. You know your child and your family best. My hope is that my insight and experience give you a feeling of connection when you need it, permission to care for yourself as you are caring for others, and some hard-earned wisdom that can help you navigate the complicated, beautiful, unpredictable journey of raising a neurodivergent child.

Prologue

Not Just Any Old Day at the Zoo

It was 1998. I was 25 years old, living in Chicago, and on a work trip to San Diego. After a few exhausting days of software training in windowless conference rooms, I was desperate for a change of scenery. Instead of catching the first flight home, I chose to stay the weekend. Just a couple of extra days, I told myself. I couldn't have known then how much that small decision would change the course of my life.

Back home, it was still winter, but here, the ocean breeze carried salt and sunlight. That Saturday, I wandered the streets and beaches of La Jolla, soaking it all in. I stopped along the cove to watch the seals sprawled out on the rocks, barking and basking in the sun as if they owned the place. Later, I treated myself to lunch at the Hotel Valencia—clam chowder by the window, the Pacific stretching wide in front of me. A view and a moment to remember.

After sleeping like a rock Saturday night, I set out Sunday morning for the San Diego Zoo. I remember the pink flamingos greeting me at the entrance, the cable cars gliding silently overhead, the polar bears plunging through the water, the elephants roaming, and of course, the famous giant pandas doing what pandas do. But none of it moved me like the sight of one small, sweet, albino koala bear.

I still don't know exactly why, but I was completely fascinated. I asked the docent so many questions: where Onya-Birri, or Ghost Boy, was born, how old he was, and which of the koalas was his mother. The sunlight caught his white fur like something I had never seen before. I learned he was the only known albino koala in captivity at the time. He was rare, so rare, and wouldn't have stood much of a chance in the wild.

He was beautiful. He was vulnerable. He was completely out of place.

I stood there longer than I had at any other exhibit, unable to look away. He seemed delicate but also quietly powerful, as if his very existence, against the odds, was its own kind of strength. I wandered the rest of the zoo, but my mind kept circling back to that little koala. Before I left, I went back to see him one more time.

Back then, I wouldn't have called myself an animal person. I didn't grow up with pets. I'd never bought a stuffed animal as an adult. But on my way out through the gift shop, I bought one: a stuffed albino koala. Something about him had touched me deeply in a way I couldn't explain.

Six years later, in 2004, I gave birth to my beautiful, one-of-a-kind son. Luke was born with a rare chromosome disorder, so rare that even today, there's only one other known person in the world with the same chromosomes. Over time, I've come to believe that Luke was the reason the little koala left such an impression on me. Ghost Boy wasn't just a moment. He was a message I didn't yet know how to read.

Like that koala, Luke is often stared at. Some people keep walking, unsure of what to say. Others linger, curious, open, and kind. Just like I had lingered that day in front of the koala enclosure, not knowing why I couldn't look away.

This book is for the lingerers. It's for the parents, caregivers, siblings, and loved ones of our beautiful, rare, and sometimes misunderstood children. It's my story of raising a boy so unique that there is no roadmap, only instinct, trial and error, heartbreak, joy, and an alarming amount of internet searching at 2 AM.

This is my love letter to the ones who don't quite fit the mold and to the messy, beautiful, real-life journey of parenting a neurodivergent child. I promise to be honest. I hope I'll be helpful. And if I'm doing this right, I'll even make you laugh once in a while—though, hopefully not at completely inappropriate times, which is when I usually do the most laughing.

I hope this book feels like a deep breath to anyone who needs one. I'm not an expert. I'm a tired mom who's made mistakes, laughed at herself, cried in the school parking lot, ate way too many pints of Rocky Road ice cream, and kept going.

Enjoy my story as I share it with honesty, heart, and a blend of tears and humor along the way.

one

EARLY DAYS—THE DIAGNOSIS

AUGUST 22, 2004. I WAS NINE MONTHS pregnant, standing at the edge of the La Jolla Cove, breathing in the salty air and watching the sunlight sparkle off the Pacific Ocean. The waves rolled in, smooth and certain, like they always had. And I remember thinking, *This is the last time I'll take in this view before becoming a mom.*

The thought filled me with wonder. It also filled me with something else, something I didn't have a name for at the time. Maybe it was fear. Maybe it was awe. Maybe it was heartburn—at nine months pregnant, it was hard to tell. I just knew that life was about to change in the biggest way. But in that moment, it was still just me, my big, round belly, and the ocean.

I was scheduled to be induced the next morning, four days past my due date. I was swollen, uncomfortable, and completely consumed with thoughts of labor and delivery. Would it be long? Would it hurt? (Of course.) Would I swear at Glenn? (Again, yes.) Would the baby have his blue eyes? Would I be a good mom? What I didn't know, what no book could have prepared me for, was that I wasn't just about to become a mom. I was about to become a different kind of mom.

My brain was a storm of baby books, packing checklists, and nursery décor. I had washed every onesie, arranged the diaper caddy 17 times, and I thought I was walking into the world that many parents walk into: the one with routine checkups, standard milestones, and sleepless nights you eventually laugh about. But I was about to enter another world entirely, one that required a different kind of strength. A world of acronyms, therapies, specialists, geneticists, and medical journals. A world that is both painfully isolating and profoundly sacred. The world of rare. The world of special needs.

But none of that had arrived yet.

Right then, I was just a mom-to-be with sore feet and puffy ankles, soaking in a quiet moment of peace before the next chapter. I didn't know that in just a few weeks I'd be studying chromosomes, battling insurance companies, and wondering if my baby would ever smile, walk, talk, or eat on his own.

And thank goodness I didn't know.

Because in that moment, looking out at the crashing waves, I was free. I had no idea what was coming, and in a strange way, that was a gift. For just one more day, I got to dream the kind of simple, innocent dreams that most parents start out with. *Will he play baseball? Will he love music? Will he look like his dad?*

I was about to meet the love of my life. I just didn't yet know how much he would change mine.

Sunday night, August 22, 2004.
"Night Zero of Parenthood"

Picture this: Glenn and I are cozied up, watching the Summer Olympics. The famous twin brother gymnasts are flying through their routines, making history. Meanwhile, my brain is off in the future, wondering: *Will Luke do gymnastics? Probably not. Track? Yes. Tennis? Definitely maybe.* My mind buzzes with visions of endless possibility until the universe sharply reminds me of the present—with my first contraction at 10:30 PM on the night before I was scheduled to be induced.

I call the on-call doc, who hears how close my contractions are and basically yells through the phone, "Get here now!"

Perfect. I know that my OB will be at the hospital at first light to swoop in and deliver Luke. Glenn loads me into the car, and off we go, just a few miles to the hospital.

It was all going according to plan... until it wasn't.

After a very uncomfortable—no, mind-blowing—hour of active labor, I begged for my "liquid relief." Enter the epidural. I thought, *I've got this. By breakfast, Luke should be here.* Spoiler alert: Mother Nature didn't read my timeline.

At 12:30 PM, 14 hours later, my doctor, calm and compassionate, exactly the kind of doctor you want as a first-time parent, declared, "Time to push." Finally! Except pushing didn't seem to come with a finish button.

Cue over three hours of effort, sweaty labor, and announcements like: "The baby's trying to come out shoulder-first... Work hard... You may be headed for a C-section." I braced for the worst, but Luke was cozy and fine on the monitors. So, I pushed on.

Over three hours later, and with no C-section required, Luke emerged. I looked at him. I looked at Glenn and saw the tears in his eyes. I felt like the richest, luckiest person alive. Love seeped out of me and into that hospital room.

Then, I crashed. Hard. I'd been awake for 34 hours, and that's nearly a day's worth of sleep deprivation in one go. So, once Luke was in my arms? Lights out. I could've sleepwalked through a marathon right after and not noticed.

At that point in my life, I was a great sleeper. I'd never pulled an all-nighter. If only I had known then that sleep was about to become an endangered species, not just for a few months but for a lifetime. After Luke was born, sleep would never really be mine again.

The Morning After—An Unexpected Turn

The next morning, a pediatrician from our practice came in to check on Luke. Everything seemed fine. He was a nearly eight-pound newborn who had made it through his first night and already had a strong, healthy cry. Then, the doctor shone a light into Luke's eyes and paused. "Luke has an eye defect," he said. "The iris in his right eye didn't fully form." My heart instantly clenched.

A *coloboma*, a rare congenital gap in the iris (the colored part of the eye) is what we were told. What looks like a "cat-eye" is really a missing sliver of iris tissue that didn't close during early development. Coloboma occurs in fewer than 1 in 10,000 births, usually affecting just one eye.

The doctor explained it could be isolated, just the eye, or part of a broader syndrome. And it could affect more than just the iris, like the retina or optic nerve, or it could even be associated with genetic syndromes. We had to wait for a full ophthalmology evaluation to know more.

I was without a smartphone then, so I sent Glenn home to do research on our desktop. The information he found was… not exactly soothing. The coloboma might be just the start. It could be part of something much larger.

That Same Night—From Fussy to Fragile

By evening, Luke was extremely fussy. I guess more so than the typical newborn because the nurse offered to take him to the nursery so we could rest for a few hours. It didn't feel right, but I desperately needed sleep.

Shortly after, there was a burst of activity. A nurse stormed into our room, lights blazing: "We noticed Luke looked slightly bluish-gray." The words echoed: "We're transferring him to the Neonatal Intensive Care Unit (NICU)." My world spun. How could this be real?

He was fine earlier, wasn't he? Glenn sprinted to the NICU for answers.

Luke had aspirated, meaning fluid had entered his lungs, and he had developed aspiration pneumonia. It's serious in newborns, particularly because their lungs are fragile, and it requires prompt antibiotics and monitoring in the NICU.

Luke ended up needing to spend four nights in the NICU on IV antibiotics and oxygen. He was also checked out, head to toe, by neonatologists, a dysmorphologist who also drew his blood for genetic testing, an ophthalmologist who confirmed his coloboma was only cosmetic (whew), and an occupational therapist. One of the doctors told me she'd bet her next paycheck that the genetic test would come back normal. That stuck with me. It sounded so confident. Luke looked typical. His exams had been thorough.

The most notable findings were an iris coloboma and a term I couldn't pronounce that essentially meant he had one unusually small toenail. That was it. And yes, of all the things to worry about, there I was searching "tiny toenail syndrome" at 3 AM in a postpartum haze. Welcome to special needs parenting, where we become experts in the most obscure medical minutiae you never knew existed.

But my instincts as a new mom told me that Luke's coloboma and unexpected aspiration pneumonia were not a coincidence. There was something bigger going on, despite all the positive news.

Luke recovered quickly and fully, and on Friday, it was time to finally bring him home. Again, we did all the things. We had Tanner, our golden retriever, sniff one of Luke's blankets before he met him. I finally got to dress Luke in his "Welcome to the World" ivory onesie. I packed his bag full of his favorite hospital binkies, and off we went with one monumental thing still lurking in the near future: genetic testing results.

The Call That Changed Everything

I remember it was a perfectly ordinary Southern California morning—a sunny, warm day that reminded me why I had moved here after that fateful visit six years earlier. I was standing in my kitchen, staring out the front window. The sunlight was pouring in—the kind of light that makes everything feel okay, even when it's not.

Luke was just over a week old, swaddled in soft blankets, and sleeping nearby. I remember how peaceful he looked. How small he seemed. How much I already loved him with a kind of intensity that scared me a little.

And then, the phone rang.

We'd been waiting for this call for over a week: the results of Luke's genetic testing. I'd tried not to obsess over it, but of course I had. Every time the phone rang, my heart jumped. Every time it didn't, I told myself silence meant good news. No news is good news, right?

The coloboma was rare, yes, but it could be isolated. A fluke. A detail. His was only cosmetic in nature, so he could go on to live a perfectly healthy life. It didn't have to mean anything. He had completely recovered from pneumonia. That was a good sign that we had a healthy baby with a strong immune system. I kept telling myself that these early road bumps meant nothing.

But deep down, I knew they did.

There was that voice inside my head that kept whispering, *There's more here*. Something unspoken, something unsettled. Luke was beautiful, alert, and already so loved. But I'd started to notice tiny things—his muscle tone, his reflexes, the way he cried. I didn't have the language for it yet, but something inside me—a mother's instinct, I suppose—was already bracing.

I answered the phone, still standing in the kitchen, Glenn by my side, staring out the front window. Again, I noticed the flawless sky. And then, the voice on the other end changed everything.

It was the geneticist. Her voice was calm, professional, and kind. But it only took a few words before my world tilted. She told me the results had come in, and Luke had a rare chromosome disorder: a partial trisomy of chromosome 14. A tiny extra piece of genetic material that shouldn't be there had attached to one of his 18th chromosomes. So small. So massive.

I was taking notes as she spoke. Words I didn't understand: Duplications. Markers. Unknown significance. Possible delays. More testing. Follow-up appointments. I wrote everything down, but when I looked at it later, it read like another language. None of it told me what I really wanted to know.

Will he walk? Will he talk? Will he smile? Will he *be okay*?

There were no answers. Not yet. Maybe not ever.

Luke's chromosome disorder didn't have a name. It didn't have a brochure or a pamphlet or a support group waiting for us. It was so rare, the geneticist said, that she had never seen another case exactly like it. There were no predictions. Just possibilities. No roadmap. Just watch and wait, and we will learn from Luke.

That was the moment we left the world of "typical" parenting behind. It didn't feel dramatic at the time. There was no sobbing, no dropping to the floor. Just a quiet stillness, like the house was holding its breath with me. I hung up the phone and stood there for a long time, not knowing what to do next.

Luke was sleeping nearby. Peaceful. Beautiful. Blissfully unaware that a phone call had just redrawn the borders of our lives.

And Glenn and I… well, we were standing in the same kitchen, staring at the same sky—still beautiful and unbothered—while our world had completely tilted on its axis.

What to Expect When... Nothing Is as Expected

I was so excited when I found out we were having a baby boy. I imagined his first step, his first word, all the firsts that were to come. Glenn and I transformed our third bedroom from a blah, beige office to the softest yellow nursery, a color we chose ourselves because it made us feel warm and safe. I arranged wicker baskets and hung the green and white gingham curtains that I made a special trip up to Orange County to buy. We were over-the-moon excited to meet Luke.

I never thought I'd be thinking of chromosomes and genetic markers. Those things sounded more like they belonged in a science textbook than the life of a baby. My ultrasounds were all normal, and Luke was growing and developing just fine in my womb. Before his diagnosis, I hadn't given much thought to milestones. They were just nice things I would capture with my digital camera and share with family. But after we found out that Luke had a rare, so very rare, chromosome disorder, milestones became my obsession. Was that a smile? Did he just lift his head? Was he tracking my finger? I started asking myself these tiniest of questions that carried so much weight. Would he ever... you name it. Walk? Talk? Play with friends? Have friends? Will he go to college? Will he get married? Yes, Luke was three weeks old, and I was wondering, daily, if he would walk down the aisle one day. Because with this uncertainty, your brain can go from "He's due in a week." to "Will he ever file taxes?" in no time flat. My mind ran ahead to every possibility, every fear, and every hope I ever had.

But the biggest worry, the one that to this day weighs heaviest on my chest, is, "Will he be healthy?" When a world-renowned geneticist and an entire team of doctors tell you that they are learning from Luke, it's terrifying, the kind of thing that's hard to wrap your head around. It's completely exhausting, in its own way.

Despite all the worry I felt and the sleep I wasn't getting, I loved every minute of being Luke's mom. Rocking him to sleep, listening to the Winnie the Pooh soundtrack or nature sounds. Feeding him, cuddling him, giving him baths. These moments became everything. I even started a journal, writing letters to him a week after he was born.

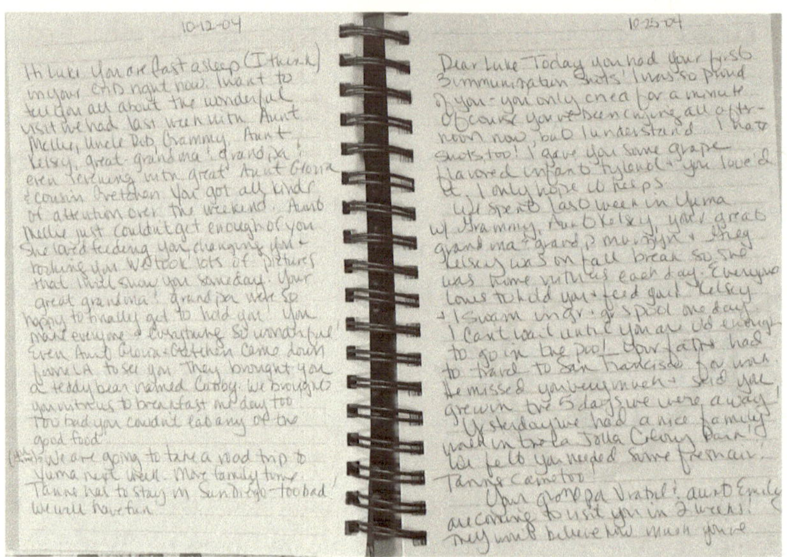

From the beginning, Luke had colic, and he cried a lot. Sometimes he arched his body in pain. Because there was so much unknown about Luke's health, I was told by a specialist that the arching could be colic, or it could be brain damage. *What?* Now I'm worrying daily about brain damage. I'm fairly certain that most parents whose children have colic aren't told that it could be brain damage. That kind of uncertainty was both emotionally draining and heartbreaking.

So much was unknown; everything was unknown. If there were an Olympic category for "Worrying About the Unknowns," I'm pretty sure I would have taken gold. What I did know was that my son was born with a very rare chromosome disorder, one that likely affected hundreds of genes on his 14th chromosome. A small, extra piece of that 14th chromosome had attached to one of his 18th chromosomes without altering it, so the real concern was the extra piece itself. Each chromosome contains hundreds of genes, any of which could influence his development and health.

Every night after I tucked Luke in, I'd go down the rabbit hole of chromosome 14. Everything I read seemed to be the worst-case scenario. And according to my many midnight searches, Luke may never get out of bed, may never smile, or may never be able to feed himself. It was terrifying, but no matter how scary it was, I couldn't stop.

I kept having this recurring dream that Luke was no bigger than my finger, and I kept losing him between the cushions of our couch. It was both terrifying and felt oddly accurate.

There were insurance battles from day one. He had spent the first four nights of his life in the NICU on oxygen and antibiotics due to aspiration pneumonia, and our insurance company at the time did not think it was medically necessary. After what felt like a zillion phone calls, letters, and appeals, they finally agreed to pay. Apparently, it takes that much to prove your baby actually needs oxygen.

Physical and occupational therapy started at Rady Children's Hospital when Luke was just four weeks old. Casi was our occupational therapist, Linda our physical therapist, and they quickly became lifelines, not just because they were helping with Luke but because seeing them was really the only time I got out of the house—aside from seeing the doctors, who didn't seem to have any answers.

Weekly appointments quickly became our routine. I called it "tummy boot camp" because those tiny workouts involved lying on his tummy (not a preferred position) and a lot of crying that could have probably broken glass. The focus was on strengthening Luke's tiny muscles, encouraging motor skills, improving balance and coordination, supporting posture, and working on sensory integration.

And then came the language lesson for me: proprioception, vestibular system, supine, prone... here we go again. Suddenly, I had to become fluent in a whole new language, learn it immediately, understand it, and use these terms daily while navigating Luke's world.

Okay, let's go!

Our therapists became so much more than just professionals; they were friends. I saw them more than most of my own family. They were hope, expertise, and the ones who helped me understand the hard stuff. Like how Luke's muscle tone issues might be due to brain differences.

My heart sank daily with worry for my little guy. But Glenn and I also celebrated the tiniest milestones, like Luke clapping his hands, which were champagne-worthy moments. It was a rollercoaster of ups and downs. When would it end? Would it ever end?

You know you're spending a lot of time at therapy when you know the ticket booth operator's schedule, how many kids he has, his weekend plans, and okay, maybe not his Social Security number, but you *do* start thinking about what to get him for Christmas.

There were so many doctors, so many appointments, and with every new concern, we were sent to see yet another specialist. Because what if? With so many unknowns, we couldn't afford to miss anything. When you have a child like Luke, a genetic mystery, everything could potentially be something. And while we were grateful for good care, we were tired of hearing, "We will learn from Luke." While I think it was meant to be reassuring, it started to feel like Luke was more of a case study than a child. After all, it was not his job to educate the doctors.

A partial trisomy of his 14th chromosome. What did that even mean? And the prognosis of "only time will tell" is not what you want to hear when you are living on caffeine and panic and could really use a dose of reassurance. But then, Luke smiled—four weeks old, and he was already proving people wrong. I had read that most abnormalities of the 14th chromosome end in a miscarriage, but there was Luke, smiling as if to say, "Don't worry, Mom. It's going to be ok."

Luke was our little miracle baby, one of a kind and full of quiet strength. He was a fighter, and deep down, there was a part of me that believed he was going to thrive. I didn't know what it would look like, but I was starting to understand what it would take to travel down this path. It was both stressful and demanding.

I remember being at a postpartum appointment shortly after Luke was born. The nurse asked how Luke was doing, and when I explained that Luke was born with a rare chromosome disorder, she looked at me with soft eyes and said, "Oh, so he's special."

She meant to be kind, but that word felt like a punch to my gut. *"Special."* What did that even mean? We're all special in some way, but right then, that word felt too simple, too packaged to explain what we were going through. It felt like a word people used when they didn't understand the enormity of the uncertainty of our grief or of the fierce love we had for Luke. Maybe she just didn't know what to say.

Luke was so rare that, early on, he ended up on the cover of a magazine out of England called *Unique*. Yes, a cover model at three years old. It was a beautiful picture of Luke holding hands with Glenn and me. Seeing it on that cover was surreal.

Reading that magazine made me realize that we weren't totally alone. There were other people navigating the world of rare chromosomes. I read about each family in that magazine, joined trisomy groups, and with the help of *Unique*, connected with a family in New Zealand who had a son, Andrew, with a similar trisomy. Andrew is a few years older than Luke, and when we looked at his photos, Glenn and I both thought, *Finally—someone who resembles Luke, who shares something rare and is a little familiar.* The best part was that Andrew looked happy and healthy and appeared to be thriving. This connection, these pictures, brought us something that no doctor or medical journal was able to bring us: hope. We've kept in touch with Andrew and his dad ever since, because when you find someone walking a similar path, you don't let go. You share stories and photos, and that reminds you that even the rarest journeys don't have to be walked alone.

I remember a visit from another "new mom" friend who clearly did not understand what I was going through as a mom to a child with a rare disorder. While she was deciding whether or not to use a wipe warmer, I was deciphering genes on the 14th chromosome. During one of our early get-togethers with our babies, she commented about how hard it was to be a new mom, and there should be a manual with step-by-step instructions on what to do. I did my best to hide rolling my eyes, and I wanted to scream, "There are! There are literally hundreds of them. Hundreds of books for you and your typically developing baby." I thought about running upstairs to grab one of the many that I had bought before Luke was born and say, "Here you go. Enjoy it while I continue to wing it with a complex genetic disorder and biology that I learned from the internet at 2 AM."

In retrospect, she was probably trying to connect with or relate to me in her own way, and being a new mom is hard no matter what. But at the time, it was hard to see that anyone else's problems were equal to my own.

Love Lesson from a Mom

To the parents who are reading this, it's okay to admit that it is hard. Really hard. It's ok to feel like some days you are barely hanging on. To have to drive to and sit through one more appointment feels like running a marathon with no training. Say it out loud. Scream it from your rooftops. Acknowledge it. Own it. It is hard. Whether it's a chromosome disorder, a physical ailment, an illness, mental health, or anything else that has shaken your world, it's hard. And it is very important to validate your feelings.

It's also okay to feel angry about all that your child is going through. You may find yourself avoiding friends who have perfectly developing kids and feel more than annoyed when they complain about how hard it is when their baby skips a nap. You may want to scream, "You have no idea!" and that is okay, too.

And let's talk about grief and getting through those hard times as a parent of a child with disabilities. It doesn't mean you don't love your child. It doesn't mean you wish they were someone else. What it means is that you're human and, sometimes, you need to grieve the picture you once held in your heart of what their life, and your life, might look like.

Not the child. Never the child. I don't want to change Luke, because then he wouldn't be Luke. And I love that kid with everything I have. But maybe, just maybe, it's okay to grieve the life you thought your child would have. Maybe it's okay to hold space for that loss and still celebrate every joyful, quirky, hard-won part of the life you *do* have.

I don't think of grief as a single emotion. It isn't neat, linear, or predictable. It's a storm that comes in waves—sometimes gentle, sometimes crashing over me with a force that steals my breath.

I have grieved the child I dreamed Luke would be and the milestones I imagined he would hit effortlessly, the simplicity of life before his diagnosis, before appointments, therapies, and constant advocacy. And yet, my grief is tangled with a love that is profound, protective, and fiercely proud.

My emotions often swirl in ways that can be confusing. There's been sadness and despair, yes, but also guilt for feeling overwhelmed, for wishing life were different, and even for feeling moments of joy in the midst of struggle. There's anger, too, at a world that doesn't always make space for Luke, anger at people who don't understand or even seem to care, and sometimes even anger at myself.

Grief can also carry loneliness. Even in a crowded room, even with supportive friends and family, the depth of this experience can feel isolating. No one else's child is exactly like Luke, and no one else's path even slightly mirrors mine. Yet, grief also opens me up to beauty and gratitude, the small victories, the quirks that make Luke authentically himself, the quiet moments that would have gone unnoticed in a "typical" life.

I don't think grief is anything that I will "get over." It's something I will always carry—though it softens, shifts and changes form. Some days, it's manageable; other days, it returns uninvited. But carrying grief doesn't mean carrying it alone. Speaking it, writing it, sharing it—these are acts of courage and love, for both myself and for Luke.

So, yes, we just jumped from me preparing for my firstborn to the emotional complexities of the grief that comes with raising a neurodiverse child. But let's be honest, if there's one thing we special needs parents are experts at, it's pivoting on a dime. One minute it's playtime; the next, it's an existential spiral over emotions, milestones, and IEP goals. Welcome to our normal.

two

EARLY YEARS—THE CHRISTENSENS & THE KID

The Power of Family

THOSE FIRST SIX MONTHS, I LIVED IN a bubble. Our world had shrunk to a simple loop: from home to Children's Hospital, then repeat. Most days, that route defined our existence.

The details blur together in a true postpartum fog. I fed Luke, changed Luke, played with Luke, attempted naps that rarely came, and pushed his stroller in endless circles around our condo complex. Nurses and social workers from Regional Center made regular visits. They were part of California's Department of Developmental Services support system, which had suddenly become central to our lives.

I read to Luke constantly, book after book, sitting with him in our glider. I felt safe in my little bubble at home, fiercely loving him and treasuring every moment of those early days. But even in that cocoon, the days were wrapped in worry and stress.

Thank goodness for my mom, Marilyn, and my sister, Kelsey. Living within driving distance during Luke's early years, they showed up again and again, hands on and ready to help. I was never too proud to accept their help, especially after I went back to work when Luke was six months old. Their presence meant Glenn and I could get away for dinner, catch a movie, or even manage a weekend escape to Las Vegas.

My mom and Kelsey were that constant in our support system, visiting regularly, loving Luke, and building their own special bond with him. My mom made up an original bedtime song that I still sing to Luke each night before we send her kisses. My mom's house was always such a warm and happy place. It was an escape from work, and there was always an overabundance of delicious food that could feed an army. I was so excited for Luke to have such a special person—his Grammy—in his life. We lost her way too early, and I still find myself grieving the moments she is not here for. The birthdays, the milestones, the everyday little joys. The memories of her and Luke will live in my heart forever.

Kelsey offered something different but equally precious: a kind, gentle love that gave Luke, and all of us, a sense of calm. She had this way of being present without being overwhelming, of stepping in exactly when needed without being asked. Her quiet strength became something we all leaned on, and Luke felt completely safe and cherished in her care.

So much family poured in that first year. My dad, my stepmom, Maura, and my little sister, Emily, who lived in Chicago, were the first out-of-town guests to arrive. I'll never forget how my dad's face completely lit up when he saw Luke, whose middle name (Thomas) honors him. My dad is the most loyal person I've ever known. His strength and unconditional love for his family are gifts that I've always known Luke will inherit. My dad loves Luke fiercely and has a very special place for him in his heart. Maura (Momo) is always kind and loving, and her visits and natural help with Luke continue today. When things with Luke get overwhelming or tense, Maura somehow knows exactly how to lighten the mood and remind us what really matters. Moments from their visit remain some of my most vivid early memories.

Emily was nine and absolutely over the moon about meeting her first nephew. She'd created a book for us, *The Christensens and the Kid*—her own illustrated story of Luke's arrival, complete with drawings of "the kid." We still reference that book today. It is safely kept in Luke's closet, and we read it often. Luke always smiles at the picture of himself in my belly, this tangible reminder of how loved he was before he even arrived.

From the moment Luke was born, Emily claimed him in a way that said, "This is my kid, too." She didn't need time to adjust or learn how to be around him. She just loved him, completely and immediately. She's proof that sometimes the most important relationships are the ones that just make sense from day one.

My sister, Melissa, who is three years younger than me, and her husband, Rob, visited early on. I later learned she was pregnant with Wil, Luke's cousin, during that visit. Wil and his younger sister, Madison, have their own special relationship with Luke—he is their 'Lukie Doodle.' Watching them together during family vacations and visits, seeing how naturally they include him in everything, reminds me over and over that love doesn't need instructions. Luke loves reading their handwritten notes, looking at photos from all the fun family visits, and the Carlsbad summer of '16 will go down in history. Their friendship with Luke will last a lifetime, and the Richters have shown us that love doesn't waver with distance.

Glenn's parents, Joan and Jack, also came out to meet their latest grandson. I have this photo of Jack holding baby Luke, and the resemblance still amazes me. You can see the family connection written right there on their faces. Jack, with his endless enthusiasm and joy for life, found his perfect match in Luke. We never thought we'd say it, but Luke is chatting just like his grandpa now, both of them able to strike up conversations with complete strangers and light up any room they enter. Joan brought her own special brand of love: steady, authentic, and unwavering. We still continue to create precious memories with her in Florida.

Glenn's brother, John, the best "funcle," is just a short drive away in LA and visits frequently. John brought this incredible energy with him, and he kept Luke looking stylish with his thoughtful gifts—whether it's the Van Halen t-shirt, the latest kicks, or a hat that makes Luke feel like the coolest kid around.

His sister, Nancy, brought her two boys, Luke's cousins, Chandler and Garrett, and we had fun playing tourists at local San Diego attractions. Nancy made visits to watch Luke play Miracle League baseball, and over the years, we celebrated many Christmases together in Carlsbad with Glenn's side of the family. Wonderful memories.

Family has always been the cornerstone of what matters to us. Family... and friends who become family.

Finding My Circle

Besides family visits, the thing that defined those first couple of years for me was early intervention. It took a little while, but eventually I was connected to an amazing group of parents—and to Nancy, an inspiring and impactful social worker who held weekly parent meetings at a local elementary school. Our kids were entertained and closely supervised in the room next door while we sat in a circle, thoughtfully led by Nancy but really driven by whatever questions, struggles, or decisions we were wrestling with as parents.

At first, I just listened. I listened to all these other parents with stories that were similar to ours—not the same, because Luke is uniquely Luke, but similar enough. Their kids had also been "identified early" by this remarkable system that serves people with developmental disabilities, a system I had no idea existed before Luke.

There we were, sitting in our circle, and I started to breathe. Really breathe. And maybe for the first time since Luke was born two years prior, I realized that I wasn't alone after all.

Sure, our stories were different, but they were also kind of the same. Our children weren't developing typically, and these parents were navigating some of the same systems I was navigating, asking some of the same questions that I was asking. Meanwhile, other parents I knew were debating whether to buy *Baby Can Read* or obsessing over the latest stroller system. *Finally*, I thought, *some people I can relate to.*

And these parents were incredible, all in their own ways. There was an artist whose husband happened to be the head occupational therapist in the school system. The mom who left her career as a social worker to stay home with her daughter. The professional stage manager and her husband who made it work as a team, balancing travel with their schedules while ensuring their daughter continued to receive her services. The mom who appeared to roll with the punches, even after her son's heart surgery as a tiny baby.

Some parents asked the brave questions I couldn't yet form. Others seemed to have mastered the art of taking life one day at a time, a skill I completely lacked. We cried together, we laughed together, and I made real connections. They were the kind of people I would choose as friends, whether I'd met them in this circle or at a coffee shop under completely different circumstances.

And maybe best of all? Luke had this super cool group of friends. These are friends he still sees today—not always often enough, but the connection will last a lifetime.

The Wagon Year

I found myself settling into the early years, even when Luke started going to a large public elementary school at the age of two. It was twice a week, half days, with the rest of his teacher time happening in our home. Sending him to a large public school so early on was tough. I remember the first day of school, when the teacher met us at the front, rolling a wagon. A literal red Radio Flyer wagon. She was picking up her students like they were library books. In went Luke, smiley as ever, and they were off, bouncing down the sidewalk like this was the most normal thing in the world.

I stood there trying not to cry. I bit my tongue so hard it bled. Something about it didn't feel right. Luke was two. TWO. I had read all the research on early intervention, and I understood the benefits, but the inner mom in me wanted to run to his classroom, snatch him up, and carry him back to my car in a dramatic, slo-mo movie moment.

Of course, I didn't do that. I stood there like a statue, with a bleeding tongue and a breaking heart. And the thing is, Luke ended up having a really rich experience in that program. He grew. I grew. We survived the wagon.

And then... he turned three.

School Days, School Days, Good Ol' IEP Days

That's when I learned about IEPs. Three innocent-looking letters that, at the time, I was sure stood for "Intense Emotional Process" because that's what it felt like.

No one warned me that I was about to enter a new dimension, a world made entirely of binders, acronyms, goals, evaluations, meetings, more acronyms, and therapy schedules that look like Olympic training plans.

I had no idea that from age three on, I'd be living inside an educational escape room where the only way out was decoding phrases like "Least Restrictive Environment" while searching "What is an SLP?" for the fourth time that week.

At the time, I was totally clueless. I still remember that first meeting so vividly, even now, almost 18 years later. It was held at an elementary school in San Diego, and I walked in, wide-eyed and trying to be optimistic. A few seasoned parents had warned me to "make sure the team had Luke's best interest in mind" and to "get everything in writing," which made it sound a little like a legal deposition. But when I walked in and the team of nine, including teachers, an assistant principal, therapists, a school psychologist, and the school nurse, were seated at a preschool-sized table and chairs, I couldn't help but feel a little of the weight lifted from my shoulders. Everyone at that miniature table seemed really nice. They smiled. They nodded. They listened. And when they talked about Luke and his assessments, it was like they actually knew him.

Later that night while picking up dinner (I remember exactly where I went and what I ordered, and yes, remembering oddly specific details like this is one of my superpowers), I started to panic.

What did I miss?

What did they really mean?

Was there educational jargon hidden between those friendly smiles?

I tried to do a mental rewind of that meeting. I had genuinely liked everyone at the table. It was basically a small village. And while they each shared assessments, goals, and services for Luke, somewhere between "gross motor delay" and "pull out speech minutes," my brain short-circuited.

I realized I couldn't remember so much that was said at the meeting.

OI, ID, SLI, SLP, SAI—turns out they stand for Orthopedic Impairment, Intellectual Disability, Speech/Language Impairment, Speech-Language Pathologist, and Specialized Academic Instruction, but at the time, they might as well have been NASA codes.

What had felt like a calm, productive meeting was now a total blur. Not because they didn't explain things—they did—but because all of this was so new and I didn't have a clue what I was doing. Sure, I had an IEP document, but I didn't understand what that meant in terms of implementing it all at school and how it would help Luke.

So, I thought, *Well, I hope all those nice people really do know what they're doing and that they'll make sure Luke gets everything he needs.*

Spoiler alert: that's not how you're supposed to feel after an IEP meeting.

My journey as a mom and advocate, trying to understand IEPs and navigate school for Luke, would take me down a winding path full of twists and turns—one that would ultimately push me to reinvent both myself and my career. And trust me, we're just getting started.

Love Lesson from a Mom

Those early months taught me that love doesn't always look big and bold. Sometimes it's quiet and steady, like the rocking chair that never seemed to stop or the same bedtime story told for the tenth time. It's okay if your love lives in a small, protective bubble for a while. Healing and connection grow there, too.

It's not weakness to need help; it's wisdom. I used to think love meant doing it all myself, proving I could handle everything. But my family showed me that real love often looks like showing up and letting others show up for you. Your village might look different from mine. Maybe it's a friend, a neighbor, or another mom who just gets it—but it counts. Every hand that helps you hold the load makes the love stronger.

Love grows in the letting go. The wagon, the goodbyes at classroom doors, the IEP meetings, all those moments that split your heart in two? They're part of the story. Every time we let go, even a little, love stretches and grows. It hurts, but it also proves how deeply we're connected.

three

THE SIBLING BALANCING ACT

LUKE'S BROTHER, EVERETT, IS FOUR YEARS YOUNGER. We didn't plan to wait that long, but I had two miscarriages in between the boys. Both were early miscarriages, and I was told by doctors they were likely due to a genetic condition or chromosome disorder.

Wait, what? So, what I'm hearing is that I've had three pregnancies, and they likely all resulted in abnormal chromosomes? It felt like a cruel joke. As if Luke's partial trisomy wasn't enough to process, now I was being told that my body might be predisposed to creating these genetic complications.

Glenn and I had our blood drawn and tested negative for any balanced translocations that could be the cause. But I was also told it's not that simple. They had only tested our blood, not all our other cells, so there could still be answers we didn't have.

Here we go again: AP Biology territory. There's a reason I never took that class in school, and now, again, I was being forced into a crash course in genetics and chromosomes.

We met with a geneticist who explained that we could do in vitro fertilization. At the time, the only option was to create embryos and then send them somewhere in Pennsylvania to test them for chromosome disorders before implantation.

That was too much. The thought of putting my sweet, precious little embryos on a plane without me and sending them across the country to be tested was just too much to process. It felt wrong—too clinical, too scary.

We decided to try again the good old-fashioned way, despite the risks and all the unknowns. And that's when I became pregnant with Everett.

The day I found out we were having another boy, I decided to surprise Glenn with the news in the most creative way my exhausted brain could manage. I bought blueberries, blue cheese, and Blue Bunny ice cream. I made dinner and dessert using all of these ingredients and asked him to guess the sex of the baby.

He got it right away. After all, it wasn't much of a puzzle. Especially since I left all the items out on the counter—even the melting ice cream.

I will add that the decision to have another child was not a small one. We had always wanted more than one, and we thought that it would be good for Luke to have a sibling. To other parents facing this decision, I want to say that there is no right or wrong choice here. There is only the choice that feels right for your family, your heart, and your capacity to manage the unknown. It's okay to grieve what's been lost, to feel fear, and to sit with uncertainty. And it's also okay to hope, to imagine the joy a new sibling could bring, and to make a choice guided by love rather than fear. Whatever path you choose, it will be deeply personal and deeply valid.

Everett was born on 08-08-08, again during the Summer Olympics, this time in Beijing, China. In Chinese culture, the number 8 is considered lucky, a symbol of prosperity and good fortune. From the very beginning, Everett lived up to that energy. He was full of life and movement.

Our couple of days in the hospital after Everett was born were pretty uneventful, with one exception. Remember the pediatrician who first discovered Luke's coloboma when he was just a day old? He was back, this time examining Everett.

Before I even had the chance to remind him that I was Luke's mom, he pointed out the creases on Everett's hands. They had a unique characteristic, he explained. Sometimes, not always, this pattern of creasing can be more typical of a child with a chromosome disorder, based on how babies fold their hands in the womb.

My heart skipped. But before the panic could take root, I stopped him. We had done early testing with Everett, and his chromosomes were normal.

We shared a moment together: me, silently relieved, and him, a kind, thoughtful doctor who had once given us life-changing news and was now part of a very different memory.

When we came home from the hospital just two days later, the phone calls started rolling in. Friends and family reached out with the most loving intentions left on our voicemail, "How are you?" "How's Everett?" "Can we bring dinner?" "Can we come by for a visit?" Each message was filled with kindness, with people who truly cared about us.

But I didn't answer the phone. I didn't return messages. And for the first month or so, I didn't want visitors. It wasn't something I had planned. It wasn't me trying to shut people out. I just… couldn't. And it took some time for me to understand why.

Because Everett was fine. We were fine. What I came to understand later was that I needed that quiet, protected space and time to simply be with my newborn and my family without the outside world rushing in. Time that I never had with Luke.

When Luke was born, we were consumed by appointments, tests, specialists, and worry. There wasn't space to savor those postpartum days, to simply hold him and breathe him in without the weight of uncertainty pressing down.

With Everett, my unconscious mind seemed to understand before

I realized what I so desperately needed: the chance to cocoon. Just me, Glenn, and our boys, wrapped in the stillness of our home. No schedules. No demands. Just us. The way it's supposed to be in those earliest days, where love is enough and time slows down just long enough to soak it all in.

And maybe that's the lesson. Sometimes what we need most is permission to pause. To step back from the noise and simply be present. To trust that caring for ourselves, and protecting that quiet time, is just as important as anything else we could be doing.

I eventually welcomed my friends and family, but I will always cherish those early days that slipped by far too quickly, yet gave me exactly what I needed.

Everett was high energy from the very beginning. Even as a baby, he would lie in his carrier, twisting his hands and feet in perfect circles over and over again. Constant movement. Perpetual motion. It was like he had this internal motor that never turned off, even when he was supposed to be resting.

I mentioned this quirky behavior to our pediatrician during a routine office visit, describing how he would make these repetitive circular motions with his hands and feet. And like clockwork, as if Everett knew we were talking about him, his little hands and feet started turning in those familiar circles right there in the exam room.

Our pediatrician watched him for a few seconds, taking in the continuous motion, the intensity of it, the way his whole little body seemed to vibrate with activity. Then, she looked at us and delivered her diagnosis in the most straightforward way possible: "That's energy. Just plain old, extremely high energy being released from his tiny little body."

No concerns. No red flags. No need for further testing or worry. Just a baby who came into this world with more energy than his small body knew what to do with, so he was literally moving it out through his hands and feet.

After everything we'd been through with Luke's diagnosis and all the medical complexities that came with it, it was refreshing to hear such a simple explanation. Sometimes a baby who moves constantly is just... a baby who moves constantly.

Everett was still in his stroller when Luke took his first step at The Getty Center in Los Angeles during a trip to see Glenn's brother, John. We assume he must have been inspired by all the beautiful art and architecture surrounding him. Perhaps Meier's stunning white travertine buildings or the carefully curated gardens provided just the right motivation he needed. Yes, another huge, champagne-worthy milestone happened smack dab in the middle of one of LA's most prestigious cultural institutions.

Everett was content to be pushed around while his big brother made history. But soon after witnessing Luke's achievement, Everett apparently decided he wanted in on this walking business as well. So, at just over 10 months old, Everett took his first step.

Let me put that into perspective: 4 ½ years and 10 ½ months. Opposite ends of the developmental spectrum, but both boys reaching the same milestone in their own time, in their own way.

It was like having a front-row seat to the most dramatic illustration of how differently children can develop. Luke's first step was a triumph over significant physical challenges, celebrated with tears and cheers and photos we'll treasure forever. Everett's first step was more like, "Oh, look at that. The baby is walking now, too," which is remarkable in its own way, but remarkable for being so beautifully typical. I will treasure both memories forever.

Two boys, two completely different journeys, both ending up exactly where they needed to be.

Early on, Luke walked with the help of his Otto Bock walker, which we were told was the Mercedes of walkers. His steps were cautious and wobbly, and he wore a helmet most of the time.

Outings were hectic. One turbo-charged child zipping around

with zero concept of danger, and the other moving slowly, purposefully, and also with... zero concept of danger.

I remember one visit to the San Diego Zoo—the same zoo where I first saw Ghost Boy—when Everett bolted, full-speed, into the dark, crowded reptile house. In a split second, I had to scoop Luke up, abandon the walker (Sorry, Otto Bock.) and go full sprint after Everett, who had the energy of a Labrador and the impulse control of, well, a labrador. Thanks to some very helpful zoo-goers, he was returned to me safe and sound.

The grocery store closest to our house had exactly one, just one, of those magical carts, the kind with two side-by-side seats where you can strap in both your kids. That cart was my holy grail. As soon as I pulled into the parking lot, I'd scan the cart corrals like a hawk. If it was there, it was going to be a good, safe, semi-sane shopping trip. If it wasn't... well, that's when things got tricky.

If the coveted cart was taken, I only had one choice: haul out Luke's Otto Bock walker. I couldn't put Everett into a regular cart alone, as he absolutely refused this option because those carts only fit one child. "Why can't I walk, too?" And if I put Luke in the cart, I heard, "Why does he get to ride?" So, we all walked and moved in slow motion. Sure, Everett would regularly take off with zero regard for aisles, shelves, or personal safety. And most of the time, I ended up scooping Luke up, ditching the walker (again), and chasing Everett around the store, just like at the zoo. Would I ever learn?

Looking back on those chaotic grocery trips, and all the days in between, I don't remember the stress as much as I remember the stories. The little victories. The fact that we showed up. Yes, it sometimes took us two hours to buy five things, and yes, we never got to the second half of the list. But we also laughed. We made memories. We bonded over popcorn and endless searches through the dollar bins, and we shared the experience of just trying to make it through the aisles without anyone escaping.

People described Everett as "wild." I remember a neighbor driving by one afternoon, smiling and calling out in a friendly, joking tone, "There's the wild child!" She meant it affectionately, but I couldn't help feeling a little twitchy, clutching my keys and silently counting to ten as Everett climbed the mailbox or something equally life-threatening.

Preschool teachers confirmed what I already knew: naps were not Everett's thing. "He just doesn't sleep," one of them said, baffled. Instead, they gave him puzzles or Play-Doh or had him "help" them with quiet tasks while the other kids dozed. He didn't nap at home either, and he had jumped out of his crib by the time he was 18 months old, like a pint-sized ninja.

Strollers? Nope. Child leashes crossed my mind more than once.

It became a daily occurrence—me, the frantic mom at the store, park, zoo, or beach, calling out his name, scanning every corner like I was in a hostage negotiation. And honestly, sometimes it felt like I was. I was also still working part time, and most days I felt completely overwhelmed.

I started to wonder, was this "beautiful wildness" just part of Everett's DNA? Or was it also a bid for attention in a house where Luke needed so much of my time? I didn't want to label him or pathologize his energy, but I couldn't ignore the question either.

The irony that Everett's typical behavior was often more exhausting than Luke's special needs was not lost on me. And of course, I felt guilty about that. How do you explain to people that the child who can walk, talk, and do everything on their own is sometimes more overwhelming than the one who can't?

I wanted Everett to know I saw him, too. That I loved his chaos. That I was in it with him. So, I made a quiet promise to myself. I would be present. I would kick the ball. Blow the bubbles. Chase him around until I dropped.

One of the beautiful things about Everett is that he sees Luke simply as his brother. Of course, he knows Luke has special needs. He knows that his school day looks different, with modified classes, speech therapy, and more support. But at home? Luke is just Luke. No disclaimers. No exceptions. No excuses. He is Everett's brother, and he gets treated with the same chaotic mix of love, irritation, loyalty, and occasional yelling that I remember sharing with my siblings.

They still have fun together. They fight over snacks. They crack each other up. And when Luke blasts his iPad at full volume, Everett doesn't go easy on him. He shouts up the stairs just like any little brother would, *"LUKE! Turn it DOWN!"* No special treatment. No awkward tiptoeing.

If Luke's on his eighth Elmo video in a row, Everett will stroll over, roll his eyes, and help him find something new. Sometimes he'll pull up animal clips or funny game videos and show Luke how to find them. Luke always lights up, not just because he's learning something new but because his brother is sitting beside him.

That's the thing. The interaction isn't "inclusive" in the staged, brochure-ready way. It's messy. It's noisy. It's real. And it's beautiful.

Between the two of them, I was exhausted almost all the time. I had one child who needed constant attention to stay safe, who required my help for every basic task, and another who demanded just as much but in a totally different way. Everett wanted me all the time, and he wanted me all to himself. I felt stretched too thin.

I'd been in pharmaceutical sales since 2000, sampling meds, memorizing side effects, and schmoozing doctors. I just couldn't do it anymore. There was too much happening at home. I was knee-deep in therapies, doctor appointments, inclusion plans, learning a foreign language known as "IEP," and constantly brainstorming new ways to help Luke communicate, connect, and thrive.

In those early years, it's all about potential. I poured everything into trying every therapy, every class, every tool, tip, and "miracle" that might help Luke reach that elusive goal: his full potential. I never stopped doing that entirely, but somewhere along the way, my focus started to shift. I stopped planning only for the future and started thinking about what Luke enjoys in the present. What brings him joy today.

And that's what I wanted for Everett, too. Not just plans and goals and structured activities but presence. I didn't want to miss him, his energy, his laughter, his ridiculous questions, his wildness because I was too busy managing everything else.

So, I tried. I really, really tried to be present.

And sometimes, trying was enough.

Love Lesson from a Mom

What I want to share is this: this, too, shall pass. Not in a dismissive way. Not like those strangers at the store who smile and say, "Enjoy every moment!" while your toddler is melting down and your cart is overflowing with dollar-bin regrets. But in a real way. In a lived-it, survived-it, came-out-stronger kind of way.

Because the truth is, someday, your kids may not need the cart, or the walker, or whatever it is you are using. Someday, you'll walk into a store and realize you don't have to scan for the "magic cart" anymore. And while you may not miss the chaos, you'll look back and see what those years gave you: resilience, patience you didn't know you had, and a deep well of love that carried you through.

That's one of the lessons I've learned as a mom. Some hard seasons pass and some don't, but they all leave us with some form of strength and compassion that never goes away.

And your effort to show up for your child is never wasted, even when it feels imperfect—and it often will. When you choose presence over productivity, when you stop managing long enough to actually see your child, you're giving them the greatest gift. You're giving them the message that they matter more than your to-do list. Some days, you'll nail it. Other days, you'll barely survive it. But the trying? The trying is always love in action.

It wasn't easy, but we got through it. Not perfectly or even close to it, but together. And now those "shopping cart days" live in my heart as some of the most beautiful messes of early motherhood.

four

Reinventing Myself, Again

I worked for a big pharmaceutical company from before the boys were born until they were almost three and seven years old. After over a decade, in January 2011, my long-running delusion that I had the "ideal working mom job" came to a quiet, exhausted end. I had been trying to convince myself for years that I could handle the balance, juggling career and caregiving like a sleep-deprived mom holding 10 grocery bags, a lukewarm coffee, and a half-written to-do list in her head, all while pretending it was no big deal. But the truth? I was tired. Really tired.

Tired of feeling that I was doing C work, at best, in every area of my life. Tired of constantly rushing Luke out the door so we wouldn't be late for school, or therapy, or the next specialist. Tired of feeling that my goal was to get to the end of each day without forgetting anything or anyone.

Yes, I was technically getting it all done, and I was doing my best to be present, but was I really living? Or was I just pushing through? Is that what it's supposed to be—just getting through it?

There was a lot of inner dialogue. The exhausting effort to convince myself that leaving my job was a rational decision. That it was okay. That I wasn't being irresponsible or overdramatic.

That this wasn't "quitting" or "retiring." It was choosing. Choosing to show up more fully for the things that truly mattered. Choosing to stop pretending I could do it all at once and do it well.

Because I wasn't just parenting. I was doing the kind of full-contact, 24/7 caregiving, therapy-coordinating, IEP-decoding, nervous-system-on-overdrive parenting that doesn't come with a lunch break. And I needed to breathe. I needed permission (from myself, mostly) to stop striving for a version of success that didn't fit my life anymore.

Leaving my job of 11 years was pretty uneventful. Following months of performance conversations, my final meeting with the district manager was unexpectedly pleasant. She wished me well. Then, someone came by and picked up my company car. Car shopping, here I come.

I acknowledge that I had the privilege to slow down and immerse myself in Luke's world, and I don't want these pages to make anyone feel guilty or excluded. Some parents are working double shifts, juggling childcare and bills, and barely catching a moment to breathe. I see you. For those who can't step away, I hope these pages offer a reminder that love and commitment show up in countless forms. Even amidst long days, crowded schedules, and exhaustion, the little moments you carve out are your own kind of presence, and they matter just as much.

It wasn't easy. I had worked hard to build a career I cared about, but when I looked at Luke, really looked at him, I knew I didn't want to miss one more minute of our life together just because I was juggling 10 balls in the air. So, I stepped away from the grind and into the chaos. Our kind of chaos. The beautiful, messy, grape-cutting, bed-pad-checking, goofy songs in the morning kind of chaos.

Now that I had more time to focus on Luke and our family, I made promises to myself. I would slow down and I would work at Luke's speed.

So, what does that even mean, "work at Luke's speed?" Well, it means letting go of the endless mental checklist constantly running in my head. Not entirely, of course—I'm still me. But it means being intentional. It means choosing to pause instead of rushing. It means walking into Luke's bedroom each morning and talking with him before immediately scanning the sheets for leaks, checking the bed pad like a forensic scientist, and calculating how many loads of laundry I'll be doing before noon. It means letting Luke move at his own pace instead of leading him around like we are on some type of morning obstacle course going for our best time.

Luke is a lover of the little things. The very little things.

Squeaky doors opening and shutting, over and over again, are a full-on concert to him. Throwing away the trash? A thrilling daily ritual. And don't even get me started on toilets flushing. He doesn't just enjoy it; he celebrates it like he invented indoor plumbing.

Who am I to rush through these moments? To him, they're not chores. They're not background noise. They're joy.

And if I'm honest, watching him delight in those tiny, ordinary things has made me see them differently, too. I used to be laser-focused on the next thing, the next task, the next appointment, the next "get out the door" panic. But Luke pulls me back, over and over again, to the now. To the door that creaks at just the right pitch. To the swoosh of the toilet and the proud *I did it* grin afterward.

So, maybe slowing down wasn't just for me. Maybe it was a way to honor the world Luke lives in, the one where joy hides in the most unexpected places, if you're willing to stop long enough to notice.

Now, instead of barking out a list of to-dos, I kiss his forehead, breathe him in, and let the morning unfold before I start to belt out *You're Simply the Best,* one of Tina Turner's greatest hits and one of Luke's favorite songs.

Mornings used to be triathlons. I'd move Luke from bedroom to bathroom to breakfast in record time. I'd wake him up, strip his sheets, brush his teeth, choose an outfit, and help with toileting. Then, there was bathing and dressing. I'd make his high-protein breakfast, make sure the iPad was charged and ready for communication, pack his lunch, always cutting grapes in halves or quarters like I was prepping for a tiny, royal tea party. And yes, I even cut his penne pasta in half. All this happened before I even had a chance to caffeinate, throw on mascara or clothes, and pretend I was ready to face adults in meetings.

I still do all of that, minus the shower, the work clothes, and the mascara, but I get to do it with more time and more heart. The dishwasher can wait. The laundry can pile up. I'll get to it later, or maybe I won't, and that's okay.

Without the pressure of being "on" for a job, we found new rhythms. Luke was almost seven years old, and Everett three, so we created silly routines. We sang songs badly. We made up dances, and Luke giggled. He'd always been a happy kid, but this? This was different. It was like he could feel my new "good morning vibes" and decided to match them.

There was now space for joy, for humor, for just being. The decision to leave my job wasn't just about stepping away from work. It was about stepping into something better. Something slower, messier, more meaningful. Something Luke and I could build together, one quartered grape and goofy dance at a time.

Leaving my job came with its own set of *What in the world are we doing?* moments. We had recently moved into a larger house that came with, surprise, surprise, a larger mortgage. We were officially a one-income family. And while I didn't want to make light of that reality, or the financial pressure it brought, I also didn't want fear to be the thing that dictated our decisions.

Because deep down, even with the unknowns, I believed things would work out. They had to.

Maybe it's a little twisted, but I think I do better when life gets hard. When the pressure's on. When I don't have all the answers (or really any of them), but I have this sense of what to do anyway. There's something in me that rises in those moments, not because I'm fearless but because I'm stubborn enough to believe there's something waiting on the other side of uncertainty.

During that season, I kept returning to a quote from a book I read shortly after college, *Simple Abundance: A Daybook of Comfort and Joy* by Sarah Ban Breathnach. I highlighted the quote back then, and I've come back to it more times than I can count. It reads:

> "Concerning all acts of initiative (and creation), there is one elementary truth, the ignorance of which kills countless ideas and splendid plans; that the moment one definitely commits oneself, then Providence moves too. All sorts of things occur to help one that would never otherwise have occurred. A whole stream of events issues from the decision, raising in one's favor all manner of unforeseen incidents, meetings, and material assistance, which no man could have dreamed would have come his way."
>
> —William Hutchinson Murray, the leader of
> the Scottish Himalayan Expedition team
> that scaled Mount Everest in 1951.

That quote has followed me through some big leaps, like when I left Chicago for San Diego at 26 with not much but a couple of suitcases, a vague plan, and a lot of naïve optimism. And again now, when I chose to leave behind my job because I needed something more. I needed time. I needed presence. I needed to say yes to the life in front of me, uncertain as it was.

And maybe, just maybe, Providence would move, too.

Right around the time I was contemplating leaving my job but before I left, Luke and I went to visit some of our dearest friends, Emma and Allison. They're sisters, close in age to Luke, who've been part of our village since the early days. Greg and Felicia are loving parents who have always welcomed our family into their home.

We've shared so many memories with their family: years of trick-or-treating through the neighborhood, pool days, birthday parties watching Allison blow out the candles in her birthday Ho Hos, and backyard BBQs with friends, most of whom were part of and understood our world. Their home has always been one of those places that feels like a deep exhale. A safe haven. A spot where the kids could fully be themselves, and so could we.

On that visit, after what was probably an endless amount of time of me asking questions about school and IEPs (Felicia has always been an amazing wealth of knowledge), she shared with me that she had recently completed an Advocacy Certificate program at The University of San Diego. She told me it was a very informative program and that she was chosen for an advocacy internship with a local non-profit that offers special education advocacy on a sliding scale to reach more families who need help at school.

I was inspired. I needed to better understand Luke's rights and our parental rights. I had to learn more about the IEP document and all those bits and pieces friends had mentioned over the past couple years about additional services—and if and when I should consent to the IEP.

Depending on who I talked to and their own IEP experience, I couldn't figure out if I should keep the IEP team close because they were my partners who shared the same goal of Luke's progress or if I should keep them close because they were "on the other side of the table."

In true Vicki fashion, I went home and signed up for the next session at USD. It started in the fall of 2010. USD is a beautiful private university, a hilltop campus overlooking the city with the most amazing Spanish Renaissance architecture. Just the smell of the buildings brought me back to when I was a full-time student, a lifetime ago.

I felt giddy, almost like a freshman in college, bursting with excitement about all the information I was about to glean. Information that would ensure Luke had the best education possible. I was about to hear from professors, attorneys, and advocates about the Individuals with Disabilities Education Act (or IDEA), learn about case law, and understand Luke's and our rights as they apply to education. Finally, real information, not just the snippets I was picking up from others—you know, the "my cousin's neighbor's kid" kind of advice that leaves you more confused than when you started.

In I walked on the first evening, armed with three different colored pens and a notebook that screamed, "I mean business!" The room was filled with other adults, who I would come to learn were fellow parents, teachers and therapists. All were there for their own reasons, but together, we would learn about special education law. The energy was palpable—part support group, part academic boot camp, with a dash of "We're all figuring this out as we go."

I listened, took notes like my life depended on it, and got to know some pretty amazing, like-minded people. These weren't just random strangers. These were my people. Parents who spoke in acronyms (IEP, FAPE, LRE) like it was a second language, a couple of teachers who had battle scars from fighting the system from the inside, and therapists who could spot a sensory issue from across a crowded room. The program consisted of six evening courses, and they flew by, which is saying something because usually anything involving legal jargon makes me want to take a nap.

The history—recent history—of special education terrified me. Like, actually kept me up at night terrified. What I can say is that I am happy that Luke was born in present times, not a few decades ago when attending a public school would not have been an option. We're talking about an era when kids like Luke were literally hidden away, institutionalized, or just written off entirely. The fact that we've come this far this fast is both encouraging and infuriating. It's encouraging because it's progress, but it's infuriating because it took this long.

One woman, Shannon, caught my attention early on in class. She appeared to be a wealth of information, the kind of person who could casually drop legal precedents into conversation like she was talking about what she had for lunch. Throughout the class, I learned that she was a former special education teacher and administrator, had attended law school, and was a trained mediator. Basically, she was what I imagined Wonder Woman would be if Wonder Woman dealt with school districts.

I thought to myself that she could be teaching this class. Heck, she appeared to know as much as the instructors. So, why would she be taking the class? Was this her idea of light reading? All I knew was that I was in the right place at the right time. This was all information I needed to understand for Luke, and having Shannon there ended up being the secret weapon I didn't even know I needed.

My baseline with special education was very low when Luke first entered school. I was starting from a "What's an IEP?" and "Wait, they have to provide services?" level of cluelessness. This class was the step that had to happen for me to become informed, to stop being the parent who nods and smiles while having absolutely no idea what anyone is talking about.

I never imagined what taking that class would lead to. My intentions were laser-focused on Luke and school, not around reinventing myself. I wasn't looking for a career change or a life overhaul. I was just trying to be a better advocate for my kid. But somewhere between learning about due process and understanding the difference between accommodations and modifications, something shifted. I was at the end of my pharmaceutical career while taking this class, and I'll add that reciting side effects and ordering samples for doctors became less and less interesting the further I got into it.

It's funny how that works, one minute you're rattling off the potential dangers of GI meds, and the next minute, you're wondering why you're pouring your energy into all of that when there are kids out there who need someone to fight for their right to learn.

What I didn't realize at the time was that I was unknowingly signing up for a complete life makeover. This wasn't just a class; it was the beginning of me becoming someone I never knew I could be. Someone who could hold her own in an IEP meeting—even the tough ones, when things get heated.

At the end of the course, I had a Certificate of Special Education Advocacy, and I was proud! Like, ridiculously proud. The kind of proud where I already knew it would be framed, and I was deciding where to hang it. I learned, and I passed all the tests along the way: legal precedents, federal regulations, state compliance requirements. I felt like a walking, talking special education encyclopedia.

I even got out of my comfort zone to stand up in front of everyone and talk about Luke and our experience with our school district. Me. The person who never felt comfortable with public speaking, especially if it was about myself. If that's not character development, I don't know what is.

During one of the final classes, our instructor dropped what felt like the opportunity of a lifetime. There was a chance to apply for one of the three open positions for that advocacy internship that Felicia had done. Three spots. Only three spots. There must have been at least 50 people in the class, all of whom had just spent weeks learning the same information I had. Any of them may have felt just as passionate as I did.

I had no idea how many people would interview, but I knew with every fiber of my being that I wanted one of those spots. No, scratch that—I needed one of those spots. It was only a few hours a week commitment, so it all felt manageable.

I felt it. Passion. The shift. Like someone had flipped a switch I didn't even know existed. I didn't understand exactly what it meant, but something fundamental was changing in me. The pharmaceutical rep who used to get excited about free lunches with doctors was suddenly thinking about becoming an advocate for kids with disabilities.

It was terrifying and exhilarating at the same time, kind of like realizing you've been sleepwalking through your professional life because someone just shook you awake. I needed this internship like I needed air. The question was, would they need me?

Long story short, I interviewed with an advocate and the director of the non-profit, and guess what? I did it. I got one of the positions! I was going to be an advocate, not just for Luke but in the community helping other families as well. Cue the victory dance and the real possibility of my resignation letter to Big Pharma.

And that's when it hit me, like a ton of bricks to the face.

The excitement calmed down, and the reality settled in. I realized what a huge responsibility this was going to be. This wasn't theoretical anymore. This wasn't taking notes in a classroom or acing multiple-choice questions about IDEA regulations. This was hands-on, real-world, "Holy crap, what have I gotten myself into?" territory.

Sure, I could learn and pass tests. Apparently, I was pretty good at that. But now, I had to actually *do* this. Not practice in some safe training environment but advocate in real meetings with real people, most of whom had way more experience than me. Like, decades more. I was about to walk into IEP meetings where seasoned special education teachers, administrators, school psychologists, and other team members would be sitting across from me, probably thinking, "Who is this newbie, and why should we listen to her?"

The impostor syndrome hit hard. What if I forgot everything I'd learned? What if I missed something crucial? What if I made things worse for the families I was supposed to help? What if someone asked me a question and I just... blanked?

What I soon realized is that perhaps the best part of this non-profit was the collaboration. Thank goodness for that because if they'd just thrown me into the deep end with a "Good luck, don't drown" approach, I would have been toast. The interns from the previous session transferred clients to us, complete with up-to-date status reports. It was like getting the CliffsNotes version of someone's entire educational journey. There were regularly-scheduled meetings where we could ask questions before heading into IEP meetings, and trust me, I had questions about everything. We got to shadow other advocates before going it alone, which was like having training wheels but for advocacy.

The consultations were in-person back then—remember when we actually met people face-to-face, giving us time to meet clients, gather information, and get in more collaboration before the meetings? It was a level of support that made this six-month internship not just survivable but successful. Of course, it wasn't without what felt like hundreds of questions and endless hours of research on my end.

I met some incredible people through this experience. And guess who had snagged one of the other two internship spots? You got it— Shannon. Of course, she did. She wasn't just a wealth of information; she was funny and so much fun to work with. Plus, she had bigger plans brewing.

Shannon told me she was starting her own advocacy business that was student-centered, with a mediation style of advocacy. She had this unique model of having two advocates with each client, if they chose co-advocacy. I loved it because it meant more collaboration with another professional, and let's be honest, two brains are definitely better than one when you're trying to decode the mystery that is special education bureaucracy.

After my six-month internship with the nonprofit was complete, I worked for her company, Pacific Coast Advocates, for about six years. And I just continued to learn. Not just the law and parental rights, though there was plenty of that, but how to take all that knowledge rattling around in my head and communicate it to an IEP team made up of individuals who all had different personalities, perspectives, and let's face it, different levels of enthusiasm for being there.

I learned that knowing the "facts" was just the tip of the iceberg. I found that the real skill was in the communication, the delicate dance that changed with each group of people and at each meeting. My job became making sure students received what they *needed* at school, while fostering the best possible relationship with the team. Because here's the thing people don't always consider: most parents are in it for the long haul. It isn't a sprint; it's a marathon that can last from preschool through high school graduation or adult transition. A positive relationship, or sometimes just the most positive relationship possible under the circumstances, is always in the family's and student's best interest. You can be right and still watch your child lack the support they need at school if you burn every bridge in the process. I've seen it happen.

So, you might ask why I left one job and jumped directly back into another when time, or lack of time, spent with Luke, Everett, and our household was my main concern. Fair question, and one my husband asked with raised eyebrows more than once. This job only required a few hours each week.

Most days, I felt like I was a stay-at-home mom who just happened to have the most meaningful part-time job in the world. A couple of times a week, while the boys were at school, I collaborated, advocated, and kept developing this wealth of knowledge that was bringing in a little money and helping Luke at the same time. It was like getting paid to help families while becoming a better advocate for Luke. Not a bad gig, if you can swing it.

I built my foundation of advocacy experience during these years with PCA. I wanted to learn as much as I could and absolutely loved our co-advocacy model. I had zero ego about being the newbie, mostly because I felt it was glaringly obvious to everyone in the room that I was the least experienced advocate there. But this is where I got that hands-on experience that no amount of classroom learning can replicate.

Even today, 15 years later, I am still looking things up and consulting with other professionals. And I'm not talking about obscure regulations buried in some manual. I'm talking about real-life situations that make you think, *Well, that's a new one.* Every student and their program is unique. Sometimes meetings go exactly how you'd expect, and sometimes... well, let's just say some meetings have provided enough material for their own book. Hmmm, book #2—lightbulb moment.

I often think back to some of my early clients and wonder what they and their children are doing today. I worked with many of them for years, watching kindergarteners grow into middle schoolers, seeing shy kids find their voices, watching some parents transform from feeling defeated to confident advocates themselves. Some of those students would be well beyond high school at this point, probably off conquering the world in their own unique ways. I worked with good families, working their butts off to make sure their child was learning and trusting me to help guide them through the maze of special education.

Somehow, six years flew by. Six years of learning that the real world of advocacy was nothing like the textbook version, that parents cry in IEP meetings (and sometimes I want to as well), that some administrators are heroes, and others... well, others are the reason advocacy exists in the first place.

My knowledge base grew, and slowly, so slowly I almost didn't notice it happening, parents from my own school district started calling me. As an expert. Me. The mom who once upon a time had never heard of an IEP was now fielding calls from parents who saw me as the person with answers.

I was proud. I am proud. But I'm still humble enough to know there's always more to learn, and I never forget the "why" behind my advocacy. It started with one confused mom trying to educate herself to make sure Luke got the best education possible. It evolved into sharing my knowledge and experience so that students in Southern California could get appropriate services and empowering parents along the way to be the best advocates they could be for their children, at IEP meetings and beyond.

Turns out, that accidental career change was the best decision I never knew I was making.

Love Lesson from a Mom

To all the parents, caregivers, teachers, and anyone else reading this book: it's okay—more than okay; it's liberating—to reinvent yourself. To discover that the person you thought you were was just the beginning. To find out that your biggest challenges can become your greatest strengths and that sometimes the scariest leap is the one that leads you exactly where you belong.

Through the years, I've shifted my mindset to not wanting easy. Easy doesn't change lives. Easy doesn't help a student who is nonverbal finally get the communication device they've been waiting for. Easy doesn't empower a mom to speak up in meetings where she used to just nod and smile. Easy doesn't give families hope when they've been fighting the system for so long that they're ready to give up.

This work is hard, messy, emotionally draining, and sometimes heartbreaking. It's also the most meaningful work I've ever done in my life. It's what I want out of my career—work that matters, challenges that make me grow, and the chance to use everything I've learned to help other families, and my own, navigate this crazy world of advocating for neurodiverse students within the special education system.

Five

Baseball, Ohana, & Everything in Between

Once upon a time, not that long ago, you might have imagined your child on the pitcher's mound, striking out batters like a little league phenom. Or maybe tumbling across a gymnastics mat, sticking the landing like a champion. Soccer, tennis, horseback riding—whatever the sport, you pictured them excelling. Medals, trophies, orange slices. The whole deal.

The good news? Many of those dreams can still happen. The experience is just different.

Luke played Miracle League baseball for ten years. He's been pushed by a U.S. Marine in a chariot at our local half marathon, and he does weekly therapeutic horseback riding. We've cheered friends on at Challenger soccer games. There are dance classes adapted for special needs. And I have a friend whose son attended an inclusive tennis camp. If you can dream it, chances are it's out there. There may be some travel time involved, or you may have to wake up before the sun, but some version of it exists.

And yes, it's different. Baseball games are two innings. Every game ends in a tie. No one's tracking RBIs. And that competitive fire you remember from your own childhood? It might not have a place here, and that can be hard. It's okay to grieve that. It's okay to miss it. Just don't get stuck comparing your child's journey to the "typical" one playing on a loop in your head.

Because this version, our version, comes with its own kind of magic.

For us, baseball was a lot about connection. The families we met through Miracle League became our community. Our team, the Mets, was known as *Ohana*, which means family. I so looked forward to our Saturdays. There was joy in the simple things—watching our kids walk, roll, or sprint (in Luke's case, occasionally drift) around the bases. We experienced high-fives, laughter, and the pure delight on their faces after making contact with the ball, even if the ball sometimes made contact with them first.

There were great friends. Big personalities. Some hilarious kids who had no idea how funny they were. And many persistent, strong-willed players who refused to let their challenges define their game.

There may not have been talent scouts at the game, but there was heart. So much heart. And that's a win you can't put on a scoreboard.

And the parents and the coaches, wow. We had a group of some of the most incredible moms and dads you could imagine. Just like at any typical little league game, they loved cheering on their kids, snapping pictures, and lighting up when their child tagged home plate. But there was something extra special about this crew. The parents, the coaches, the buddies... they weren't just part of a team. They were part of our family.

Luke's buddy, Steve, was one of those rare people who made a lasting impact. A retired San Diego police officer, Steve heard about Miracle League on a radio ad while driving one day. He signed up soon after and eventually became Luke's buddy for many years. He was more than someone who helped him around the bases. He taught Luke how to tag home plate and then wave proudly to the crowd like he'd just won the World Series.

When we lost Steve to cancer, it was one of the saddest times in my life. I still tear up when I think about him, not just because I miss him but because he wasn't just a Saturday volunteer. He was our friend. Luke's friend. He came to family parties. He showed up for Luke and the team. He was part of our story. He was family.

This Is Not a Drop-Off Party

Some of my favorite memories from Luke's childhood are the birthday parties. We usually threw ours at a local park, and I always went all in. One year, I ambitiously tried to make a blue train cake—a blue train that looked like it hit a pothole on the way to the park. Another year, I decided pudding cups and mini muffins would be the dessert of choice. Why? Honestly, I think it's just what Luke was into that week. I gave it a lot of thought, brought everything but the kitchen sink, and still forgot napkins.

There was the year the kids took turns racing down a grassy hill in a wagon with "Uncle John"—no regrets, minimal injuries. One year, we even booked a music therapist, whose car broke down en route, so we improvised with Luke's bongos and a whole lot of rhythm.

We also attended lots of parties at friends' homes, pool parties (translation: at least one of us was getting soaked), roller skating parties (my personal favorite because I can still skate backwards like it's 1986), and yes, bounce houses. I'm still recovering from the time Glenn took one down with him inside it. Suspicious? Yes. Memorable? Absolutely.

And then, there was the infamous party at Misty's house. Misty has the energy of three humans and had graciously opened her home to a group of kindergartners, most with special needs. Just as things were ramping up, one mom casually asked, "What time should I come back to pick him up?" Misty blinked, smiled, and shouted, "This is NOT a drop-off party!" I still laugh thinking about it. Picture a house full of fast, impulsive kids, half of them expert escape artists, and she thought she was just going to leave?

Once Everett came along, and I started attending "typical" birthday parties, I realized something. All that chaos? That beautiful, bonkers energy? It was typical. Beautifully, hilariously typical—and just a little terrifying.

And by the way, when we throw Luke's next birthday party, I want to be clear: it is still NOT a drop-off party!

Potty Parties

Since we're on the topic of parties, let's talk about the least fun one of all: the potty party.

We spent more than one spring break during Luke's early years throwing these so-called "parties" with therapists who swore they'd make progress on toileting. There's a reason we did this over more than one spring break, and it's called "no progress."

Let me be clear: a potty party is no party. In fact, I think agencies should be legally banned from calling it that. It's false advertising. There were no balloons. No bounce houses. No roller skates or party favors, unless you count a pack of pull-ups and a timer set to buzz every 15 minutes.

So, what is a potty party?

While your friends are enjoying spring break in Hawaii, Palm Desert, or even just relaxing at the park, Luke and I are camped out in our upstairs bathroom. For five straight days. With our ABA therapist. Or sometimes one of her brave colleagues because even she couldn't stomach five full days of this.

We load Luke up with all his favorite drinks and then sit... and wait. The theory is simple: track intake, record output, unlock the mysteries of the bladder, and boom—progress! We had charts, schedules, and reinforcers. We were READY.

But here's the thing: Luke has never cared about schedules. Or data. Or science.

He could drink the exact same beverage, the same amount at the exact same time, and one day he'd pee an hour later; the next day, three hours later. Sometimes not at all. "He's stumping us," they'd say. "We've never seen this before." Sound familiar?

Another spring break, down the (toilet) drain. No progress, just a very clean upstairs bathroom and an urge to go literally anywhere else. Maybe next year we'll try the beach.

Enough Is Enough, or Is It?

Again, here's that deeper truth. When your child is behind on developmental milestones, you'll do anything to help them make progress, even if it means spending your precious vacation holed up with juice boxes and a laminated pee log. Your head gets full of "what ifs." What if we just try a little harder? What if one more therapy session makes the difference? What if we read one more book, buy one more gadget, try one more therapist?

Because when they're little, the possibilities still feel wide open. Every effort feels like it could be the thing that helps your child unlock something new. And you'll try all of it because sometimes that's what love looks like.

But somewhere along the way, a new thought sneaks in: what if the most important thing I can do is enjoy my child?

There's a fine balance between doing everything you can and still making room to laugh, to breathe, to just be. Trust me; these moments matter. Because your child, with all their unique needs and their own beautiful path, is still a kid. And you're still their parent.

The hard part is that there's no clear answer as to how much is too much.

No user manual. No flashing sign that says, "You've officially done enough! Take a nap." There's just you, trying to do right by your child, sorting through a million expert opinions, late-night internet rabbit holes, and that little voice in your head whispering, *Maybe if I add just one more therapy session each week...*

You want to give your child every chance. Every opportunity. Every ounce of possibility. But where is the line between dedication and depletion? Between support and burnout? That line can be blurry. And it seems to change, often.

Some days, you'll push through another hour of therapy with your game face on. Other days, you'll skip it and eat popsicles in the backyard because that's what you both need. And both are okay. That's parenting a child with complex needs. It's equal parts strategy, intuition (your gut), and survival.

So, if you're sitting there wondering, *Am I doing enough? Am I doing too much?*, you're not alone. I've been there. Most parents have been there.

Love Lesson from a Mom

The truth is, the fact that you're even asking yourself those questions already says so much about you. It means your heart is in the right place. It means you're paying attention. It means you care enough to reflect, to second-guess, and to keep trying.

That matters more than you realize. Parenting isn't about getting it perfect. It's about showing up, again and again. It's about being willing to grow alongside your child, to learn from mistakes, to pivot when something isn't working, and to celebrate the tiny wins no one else might even notice.

You might not see it in the day-to-day grind, but your child feels your effort. They feel your presence. They feel your love. That's the stuff that builds security and trust, the foundation that matters far more than whether you picked the "right" therapy, signed up for the "perfect" activity, or got every detail just so.

Always remember that your path may be different, but it's not less.

So, take a deep breath. Remind yourself: *I'm here. I'm trying. And that alone is enough.*

And parents, be safe in those bounce houses.

six

THE BANANA BLESSING &
THE CURSE OF THE CARROTS

I KNOW WHEN TO COUNT MY BLESSINGS. That isn't me being sarcastic. Yes, I do things daily, especially now that Luke is an adult, that most parents haven't done since the toddler years. Toileting, bathing, full-contact support for almost everything. But here's one solid win: Luke loves food. Like, *really* loves it. Enthusiastically. Consistently. With passion!

Over 20 years of eating, and the only thing I've ever seen him spit out in protest? Those dried seaweed snacks. And honestly, I agree. They smell like aquarium water.

Now, there are foods I won't give Luke. Not because he wouldn't like them (he would) but because I'm terrified he'll choke on them due to the low muscle tone in and around his mouth. Think tough meats, raw veggies, or anything that requires a jaw workout. Baby carrots? The ultimate villain. They sneak onto every school lunch tray and kid's meal, and Luke adores them. But trust me, those little orange grenades are dangerous. I cook his carrots into a state that can only be described as "pre-digested mush." And he still loves them.

We keep an anti-choking device in our pantry, right next to the fire extinguisher. For anyone not familiar, it is an emergency handheld device designed to help clear airway blockages when someone is choking. Glenn and I have read the instruction manual so many times we could probably use it blindfolded, underwater, while holding a banana.

Speaking of those, Luke is obsessed. He asks for a banana no less than 10 times a day. Ripe, underripe, banana bread, banana oatmeal, bananas on bananas. At 2 AM, I've searched "Can you get hyperkalemia or too much potassium from so many bananas?" Spoiler: unless Luke starts eating 400 bananas a day, he's good.

The rest of us in the house? We've officially boycotted bananas. We've scrubbed banana goo off couches, clothes, countertops, car seats, and even the dog. We are a banana-free people. But for Luke? Bananas forever.

He also loves fruit, soft veggies, oatmeal, fish, vegan cheese (disgusting, but fine since he's lactose intolerant), turkey roll-ups, eggs, and lactose-free yogurt. There's always something I can offer him, and he's always thrilled. No picky eater meltdowns here, just grateful food joy.

Now, I'm not claiming victory as a food supermom. Everett would live on fast food if left unsupervised. So clearly, this wasn't a strategic parenting win. It's just Luke. But it's a win I'll take.

And about that lactose intolerance; we figured that out when Luke was two. Up until then, we thought he had asthma. So many unnecessary breathing treatments, and turns out it was that damn dairy!

So, being able to cook, bake, and help Luke enjoy his meals has been one of our unexpected blessings. Even now, at 20 years old, his meals are often the highlight of our day.

I know that's not the case for everyone. Many families struggle with food. Every texture, every smell, every new bite becomes a battle. There are endless food therapy sessions, worries about calories and nutrition, and fears about what might happen if your child just won't eat. I know this.

I wish I had advice about food that could really help, but there are experts for that. What I can offer instead is this: find joy wherever it shows up. Maybe your child lights up on car rides. Maybe it's walking the same route through the neighborhood every single day. Or maybe the sweetest part of their day is simply being home, in their safe place, with you. Lean into those moments. Those small joys—the ordinary, repeated, almost invisible ones—are often the very thing that carry me through the hard times.

Sleep Is for Amateurs

Oh, those early days of colic. The crying, the arching, the moment you think they've finally drifted off only for it to start all over again. I think all parents enter a state of extreme sleep deprivation in the beginning. Round-the-clock feedings, living in a fog, floating through that newborn bubble. I remember going to a holiday party when Luke was four months old and catching a glimpse of the San Diego skyline, something I used to see almost daily in my pre-mom life, and thinking, *Whoa, hello outside world. I forgot about you.* Except for therapy, of course. It was surreal. It hit me then just how much my life had changed.

For most parents, those early days start to ease up eventually. You begin getting out more. Maybe you go back to work. The baby starts sleeping through the night, and that means, miraculously, you may, too. You start to feel human again. There's light at the end of the tunnel, and you think, *Ah, yes. We weren't meant to sustain this kind of madness long term.*

But then, sometimes the tunnel just keeps going.

For some of us, the sleep deprivation doesn't magically go away. The weeks turn into months, and the months into years, and your child still isn't sleeping through the night. Maybe it's because of medical needs that require overnight interventions. Maybe their brain just isn't wired for sleep-circadian rhythm. In our case, it was overnight accidents—wet clothes and sheets that needed changing. For a long time, I told myself this would pass. Just a little longer. We'll get there.

And then, you hit the stage where you realize, *This may never change.*

We tried everything. Every overnight diaper on the market. We doubled up, tripled up. If someone had suggested bubble wrap, I might have tried that, too. Still, the leaks. It's been a while since I took physics, but I genuinely cannot understand how the diaper remains dry, yet everything *else*—pajamas, sheets, stuffed animals within a 10-foot blast radius—gets soaked. It defies science.

Eventually, you stop overthinking everything and start investing in really good laundry detergent. You get used to stripping the bed in the middle of the night, swapping pajamas, whispering, "Please go back to sleep," to a now wide-awake child. And somewhere along the way, you realize, sleep is for amateurs. The pros know how to function on four hours and a cup of coffee that went cold hours ago.

Then one day, you're driving, half-awake, listening to NPR, and an expert starts talking about new research that links long-term sleep deprivation to an increased risk of dementia. Great. Just what I need. Now, in addition to the sleep I'm not getting, I get to worry about my brain slowly turning to mush.

And the spiral begins. What if I can't take care of Luke one day? Will Glenn have to take care of both of us? What if *he* gets dementia, too? After all, he's sleep-deprived right alongside me. What about Everett? What kind of future are we handing him?

Suddenly, I'm not just worried about bedtime accidents or how many diapers to layer. I'm worried about generations of exhaustion. What if sleep, or the lack thereof, becomes a family legacy?

Love Lesson from a Mom

I guess my message is this: try to find joy in the everyday moments. Sometimes it's in the foods your child loves, the little rituals you share, or the quirky, ordinary moments that make life richer. Loving your child doesn't mean your life looks the way you imagined. It means embracing who they are and celebrating the wins, big and small, that show up along the way.

I wish I had all the answers to this sleep stuff, but I can share what I've learned along the way. First up, try to go to bed a little earlier. Even if, like me, you've turned your quiet, dimly lit house into your personal temple of peace, sometimes you have to choose sleep over savoring the silence.

And here's the golden nugget: learn to take productive naps. If you take away one thing from this book, let it be how to take the perfect nap. This is for people who usually wake up more tired and, honestly, way crankier than before they took the nap.

Here's my 10-step, foolproof nap recipe that I heard on a podcast years ago. It works.

1. Find your nap spot—bed, couch, wherever. Get it ready. Blinds shut. Kids, pets, and spouses *out*.

2. Make sure everyone knows: "Do not disturb for the next 30 minutes."

3. Turn off phone notifications (yes, even that one).

4. Brew 6 ounces of strong, black coffee.

5. Drink it quickly.

6. Lie down with a blackout eye mask on.

7. Think calming thoughts. Birds chirping or frogs croaking works for me.

8. Set an alarm for 30 minutes.

9. Nap, or just rest. Don't pressure yourself to sleep, and you'll probably doze off.

10. Wake up right when the alarm goes off.

I know, I know, you're skeptical. I used to be the worst napper ever. My family begged me not to nap because I'd wake up even more irritable. But this little trick works. It has something to do with caffeine blocking adenosine receptors (science stuff), then kicking in right as you wake. Whatever it is, just try it. Trust me. You're welcome.

seven

What Does Inclusion Really Mean?

(Spoiler—It's Not Just Letting Him Sit in the Back of the Class)

I'll start by saying that overall, Luke's experience with inclusion at school has been good. He has had some amazing teachers, instructional aides, and peers along the way. He went to an elementary school with a strong sense of community and compassion, and he was in a general education classroom for a good part of the day. He loved being there, especially the read-alouds, his classroom buddies, and the dog training clicker the teacher used during reading groups to sound out syllables. A literal dog clicker. And yes, we still have one. We bust it out when we really need to get his attention.

We moved to a new school district when Luke started first grade.

Kindergarten in our first district had gone relatively smoothly, Luke loved his general education class, and we felt good about his placement. He was in a special day class as his primary setting, but he spent nearly half his day with his neurotypical peers. So, of course, we assumed the transition to the new school and district would go just as smoothly.

Then I made an early phone call to the program specialist in our new school district. That's when my heart did a full somersault.

When I asked about inclusion, she cheerfully said, "Oh, yes! Every Friday afternoon, the special education kids hold hands and walk through the general education classes."

Wait, what? A parade? Were they on display? Was Luke going to be trotted through campus like a circus act? Had I moved to another planet? It was only a 25-mile move.

I cried.

And then, I pulled myself together and told her, firmly, that we were going to stick to the plan that was working. Luke was going to be an actual student in the general education classroom, and he was going to be recognized as a student in that classroom, even if he wasn't there all day.

She agreed... with a lot of hesitation.

I was never witness to the so-called "parade," and Luke ended up having a solid year in both his special education and general education classes. He was happy. He was engaged. The teachers were warm and capable.

In fact, the year went so well that I asked the principal if Luke could repeat first grade just to stay with his gen ed teacher one more year. And the principal said yes.

The elementary years are, in many ways, the easiest years to include kids. Everyone is learning to read. School is still exciting and new. Social hierarchies haven't fully taken shape, at least not in those early grades. Kids are naturally more open to differences. They're learning about how we're all the same in some ways and different in others. And teachers? Well, most of them are excited to shape young minds. Most. Not all. We definitely had some who didn't quite buy into inclusion, and those years were harder. But they weren't impossible because everyone on

"Team Luke" made sure he was included in all his classes. Meaning, his work should hang on the wall like every other student's, and his name tag should be on his desk on back-to-school night. I met every teacher, gave them as many tips as they would listen to, and let them know I was always available to talk if they had any questions. Some of the teachers did have questions. "What is the best way to motivate Luke?" "What is his favorite snack?" "Can he have snacks?" "How do we get him to focus when he gets distracted?" I love this type of communication, and it usually helps.

We had one bad year—well, part of a year—in those early school days. The district brought in a new teacher from out of state to better support a particular student in Luke's special education class. I was impressed that they did a national search. I thought, *Wow, they must really want the best of the best.* Let's call her Lisa.

I welcomed Lisa on day one with open arms and a bag of school supplies. I told her to let me know if she needed anything. At this point, I was more than a parent. I had been advocating and helping other families for over a year, and I wanted to build bridges for Luke to help him thrive. The first few weeks seemed fine. Or so I thought.

But then, I started to hear things. Whispers. Long lunches. Aides doing all the work. Lisa, MIA. I started paying closer attention.

One day over my own lunch break, I dropped by unexpectedly because I'd forgotten to send some cream Luke needed for a minor rash. I figured I'd find him at the lunch table or out at recess, his favorite part of the day. Playing catch, swinging, maybe hanging out at the buddy bench like the social butterfly he was. These were the golden moments of natural inclusion.

I headed to the lunch tables, no Luke. I walked over to the playground, still nothing. But there were plenty of kids from Luke's general education class, so I knew I hadn't gotten the time wrong.

Then, it hit me: *Check the special education room.* I walked in, and my heart dropped.

There they were. All the kids, sitting in the dark. Watching some random movie. Six or seven students and one adult. That's it. Luke, who was supposed to have 1:1 aide support, had none in sight.

And there he was, sitting sweetly at a table with a smile on his face because that's just who Luke is. He didn't realize how wrong this all was. In front of him was his Ziploc bag full of cut-up grapes. Someone had remembered the grapes... but forgotten to *open the bag*. Luke couldn't open it by himself.

When he saw me, he lit up, reached out his little hand holding the unopened bag, and in the sweetest, most trusting voice said, "Help."

I opened the bag so Luke could eat his grapes.

I was furious.

But there was no one to direct the fury at. The only adult in the room was caring for a medically fragile student, and I could see she was equally frustrated. She was doing her job to keep that child safe. But the result was that Luke and several other students were essentially left unattended.

Remember, Luke has low muscle tone in and around his mouth, so I constantly worry about choking. The fact that someone handed him grapes in a bag he couldn't open, left him unsupervised, and called it "lunch" is... well, you can imagine the rage bubbling just under the surface.

I took a few deep breaths—more than a few. Somehow, I kept it together and decided that we needed to get out of there. Immediately.

As we were leaving, I saw the principal. I calmly (okay, *calmly enough*) let her know that I had just walked into a classroom where multiple students were unsupervised. I told her the situation was not only unsafe, it was discriminatory. I said Luke wouldn't be coming back until we had a sit-down with the school and made some big changes. And I would personally be inviting the Director of Special Education and the Superintendent.

That got their attention.

Later that day, I got a phone call. Big changes were happening the next day. Lunchtimes would now be staggered so students could be properly supported. Luke would have his 1:1 aide with him at lunch and recess. He would eat with his peers at the cafeteria tables and play alongside them on the playground—you know, like his IEP already said he should be doing.

I simply said, "Okay. I'll be stopping by periodically to make sure that's happening."

I was told that was not school policy.

I asked, "Is keeping my son segregated from his general education peers, left unattended and unable to access his food school policy?"

Silence.

Then, "I'll make myself available to escort you when you feel it's necessary to stop by."

Thought so.

It was a tough year. I mean, sleepless-nights-stress-induced-hair-falling-out kind of tough.

It was the only year I brought an attorney to Luke's IEP meeting.

I fought, and I use that word deliberately, for a reading curriculum that the entire IEP team had agreed he needed: a sight word-based reading program. Why? Because Luke, despite his many delays, had a phenomenal memory. We're talking "scored in the average range when compared to same-aged peers" kind of memory.

When you get a report like that for a kid who's scoring below the first percentile in almost every other area, you run with it.

Maybe he couldn't decode, but this kid had memorized hundreds of words. Edmark was perfect for him. Everyone agreed, in writing, at the end of second grade.

Then came 3rd grade. New teacher. New problem.

No Edmark.

"Oh, it's been ordered," they said. "It should arrive soon."

Weeks went by. Nothing. I started asking, politely at first, every few days.

Eventually, I asked who in the district I needed to contact to check the purchase order status. Maybe I could help speed things along.

Crickets.

Let's be honest. It hadn't even been ordered.

So, after many deep breaths, I sent an email. A well-worded email that basically said, *If Luke doesn't have the Edmark program by Friday* (it was Monday), *I'll be filing a complaint with the Office of Civil Rights.*

I already had the number saved in my phone.

Edmark arrived on Thursday.

But wait, it gets better.

The program showed up, but was it being used? Nope. I was told Luke had started it, but a little bird, bless her, let me know otherwise. Edmark was collecting dust.

So, I called Edmark myself.

"Hi! Quick question: is there a way to print a student's usage and progress report?"

"Absolutely!" the customer service rep replied. "It's one of the best features. You can track everything!"

You know what I did next.

I emailed "Lisa" and asked for Luke's progress report. I cc'd the principal and the district.

Let's just say they were less than enthusiastic about providing it. But after multiple follow-ups, they finally sent it.

Luke had spent a total of **20 minutes** on the program in **six weeks**.

Her excuse? "We are having computer issues."

Sure, they were.

Then came the kicker.

When she finally started using the program, or said she was using it, I was told Luke was struggling with Lesson 5 and couldn't move forward.

Another bird whispered the truth: *Lisa was taking the tests for him. And failing them. On purpose.* To prove her point that Edmark wasn't right for him.

So, let's recap. Not only was she withholding the program he loved, she was actively sabotaging his success with it.

Enter attorney. Emergency IEP meeting. No more games.

The outcome? Luke was granted compensatory education in the form of after-school tutoring sessions, several days a week, with an aide who actually used Edmark.

About six weeks later, that aide, unaware of all the drama, proudly handed me a certificate.

"Luke Christensen has passed Lesson 75." Yes, 75.

This child that they said was struggling to get through Level 5 had blown through the program and loved every second of it.

Of course, I immediately emailed a photo of the certificate to everyone involved.

More crickets.

So, here's the takeaway. We. Have. To. Pay. Attention. Even in a strong district. Even with a solid IEP. Even when everyone seems supportive. Because many of our kids can't tell us when something's not right. Luke couldn't say, "My teacher's not using my reading program," but he did show signs. He started quivering his chin in the car on the way to school. He didn't want to go. And Luke loves school. He trusts just about everyone.

I had to get creative. I made visuals with photos of his teachers and aides and asked him, "How does this person make you feel?"

His answers were consistent. I took a video of Luke using the pictures and sent it to the principal and special education director. Per my request—scratch that, per my demand—he was pulled from that classroom. We didn't know exactly where he would go next, but we knew one thing for sure: as far as Luke was concerned, Lisa was done.

And let me say this: our district is excellent overall. This was an anomaly. Luke is almost 21 and has had a solid educational experience filled with exceptional teachers, therapists, aides, and staff.

Belonging

That year tested every ounce of my patience and strength as a parent. But it also opened my eyes to what true inclusion really means and what it looks like when it's missing. Because inclusion is about being seen, supported, and truly part of the community.

Let's start with what inclusion is not. It's not just physically being in a general education classroom. But honestly? There are still schools where even that first baby step is considered a win. So, yes, we've made progress, but we still have a long way to go.

Inclusion is about belonging.

Luke was my first child, and Everett came along four years later. So, when Luke started school, I had no prior experience. Now that I've been through it again with Everett, I see it more clearly. When a child with special needs is included in a general ed classroom, even part-time, parents should have the same expectations as every other parent in that room. That's the bar. Not "Isn't it nice that he gets to sit in here?" but "He's a full member of this class."

Start on day one. Your child should be welcomed, known, and valued. Their name should be on the class roster. They should have a desk or a cubby or a hook with their name on it—whatever all the other students have. I'm not asking for red-carpet treatment here, but your child should feel like part of the classroom community from the start.

Parents, talk to your child's teacher ahead of time and ask which classmates might make great peer buddies. Trust me, there are always a few. And those relationships can make a huge difference. Buddy them up. These little things help create a sense of connection and comfort, and they're great for everyone involved.

And speaking of classwork, let's talk about differentiation. Does the work need to be modified? Who's doing that? What supports will your child need to access the curriculum? Visuals? Hands-on activities? Movement breaks? Chances are, some of these tools are already being used in class anyway because, let's face it, all kids learn better when they're engaged with visuals and movement.

These supports should be in place on day one, which means they should have already been discussed and written into the IEP.

What we're really talking about here is meaningful participation, not just being in the classroom but being part of the class. Every student, including yours, should be engaged in class assignments in a way that makes sense for them. This is where modified work, visuals, assistive technology, and a whole lot of flexibility come in. Their work may look different, but it's still connected to the class topic, and it should be valued just like every other student's work. Participation doesn't have to look a certain way to matter.

All students deserve to be called on, encouraged to contribute, and given the time and space to respond in the way that works best for them, whether that's with speech, an AAC device, picture cards, gestures, an epic facial expression, or belly laughing—the kind where you hope they remember to inhale and it seems like too much for their little bodies to handle. Luke's specialty, by the way.

Your child should be included in the everyday rituals that create community: morning meetings, job charts, being the line leader, and running notes to the office. Let's be honest, that office errand? A rite of passage. If your kid isn't getting the chance to deliver an envelope with mysterious contents to the school front desk, we have a problem.

And you, dear parent, can absolutely volunteer to be a room parent. It's a daunting task, I know. Coordinating 24 kids' Halloween party snacks and trying to come up with new, healthy snack ideas that are gluten-free, allergen-free, low sugar, organic, dye-free, and come in reusable, recyclable packaging can be a headache, but if you're up for it, more power to you!

If you work or simply do not have the mental space to volunteer, that is ok. Your presence, love, and the little ways you show up for your child everyday matter far more than any party planning or classroom task. Volunteering is wonderful, but it's not the measure of your dedication or your worth as a parent.

True inclusion also shows up outside of the classroom. Ask the teacher to connect you with the parents of those amazing peer buddies (you know the ones—if not, find them). And suddenly, playdates and park meetups could become part of your life, too. This is the beginning of community inclusion.

This is you, standing proudly and saying to the world, "This is my child. They will be seen, heard, included, and valued just like anyone else."

Remember, inclusion doesn't happen overnight. It takes patience, persistence, and sometimes trial and error, but each small step counts.

And just when you finally start to feel like you're getting it, that this wild, winding road called school might be navigable, when you've figured out how to communicate with teachers and staff without crying (at least most of the time), when the baby steps feel like they're finally leading somewhere, when your child has found their rhythm and maybe even "their people"... BOOM. You hit middle school.

Middle school.

Cue dramatic music.

Hormones. Social hierarchies. No more recess because now, apparently, it's "cool" to just stand around and stare at your phone after lunch. Way more students. New teachers. New classrooms. And surprise, students and families who haven't had the benefit of the last few years of your personalized "my child may do things differently, but they belong here just as much as anyone else" TED talk.

Did I mention hormones?

It's a reset in so many ways. The rules change. The vibe changes. Suddenly, everything feels less warm and fuzzy and a little more chaotic and unfamiliar.

So yes, we're going to take a pause on school here. Because as we head into the teen years, there's so much more to unpack. School still matters, and we will come back to it, but so do a million other things, such as growing independence, medical decisions, friendships, puberty, advocacy in a bigger world, and what it means to raise a young adult who is still very much your child.

Love Lesson from a Mom

We must stay vigilant: asking questions, noticing small changes, and ensuring children have a voice through whatever means necessary, whether that's technology, thoughtful questioning, or creative communication tools.

Never stop advocating because our kids deserve nothing less.

That experience I had when Luke was in elementary school knocked the wind out of me. I had already completed my Certificate in Special Education Advocacy from the University of San Diego. I knew the law. I understood our rights. I was even helping other families navigate their own IEP journeys.

It showed me exactly why even the most informed, prepared parents often need an advocate.

Because when it's your own child, when it's your son sitting in that classroom without the support he needs, it's not just strategy and paperwork. It's not just procedural safeguards and timelines. It's personal. Deeply personal.

There were real sleepless nights. I wasn't the calm, composed professional at Luke's IEP meetings. I was his mom—a mother trying to stay composed while fighting with everything she had.

And that's the truth. You can know the law inside and out and know exactly what your child needs but still be overwhelmed, rattled, emotional, and raw when those needs are being ignored.

Advocates or friends who understand the system but aren't the ones living it can bring that steady, outside voice when your heart is breaking. They can say the hard things when you're too exhausted. They can hold the system accountable when you're just trying to hold it together.

That's what I've learned. And it's why I will always encourage other parents, especially those navigating tough seasons, to lean on help when they need it. You shouldn't have to go it alone.

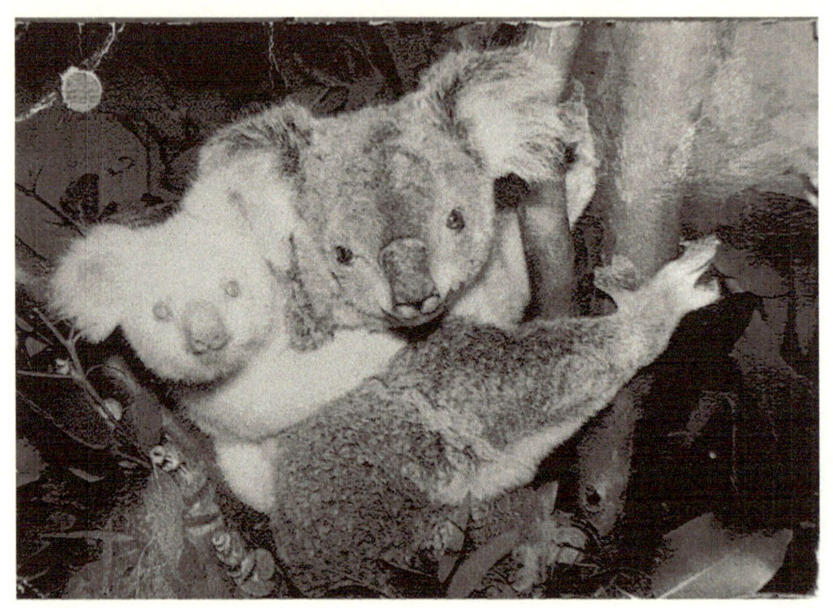

Onya-Birri "Ghost Boy"

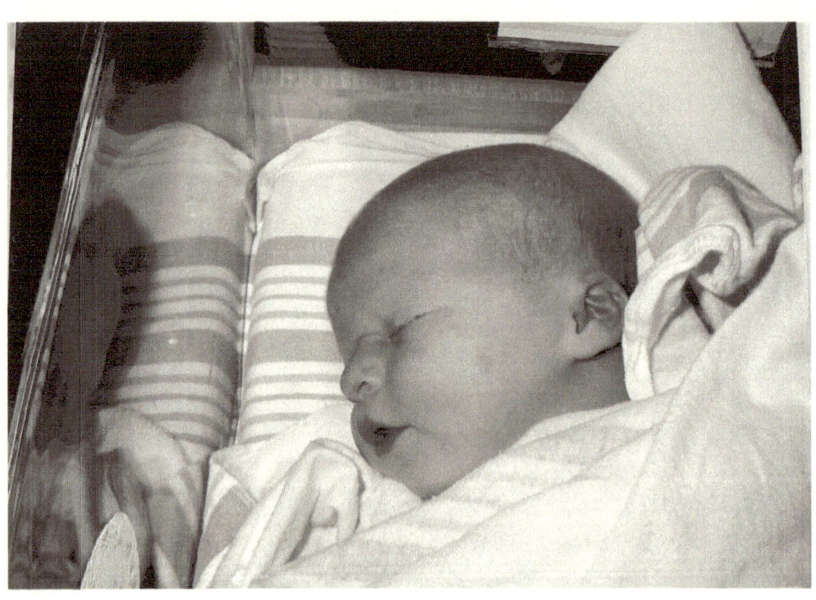

Luke 8-23-04

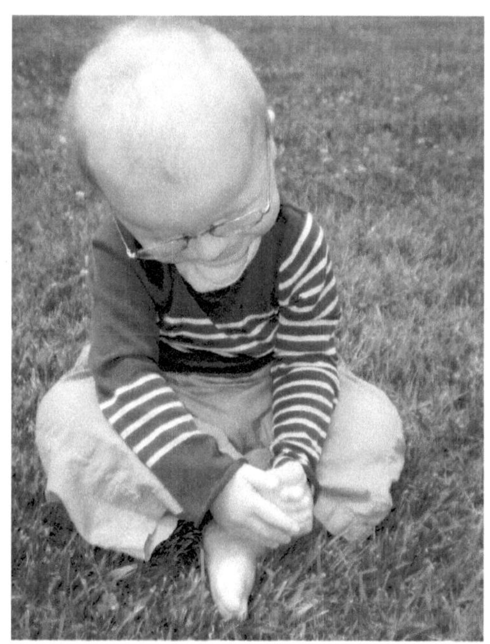

Luke discovering his toes while wearing his new glasses

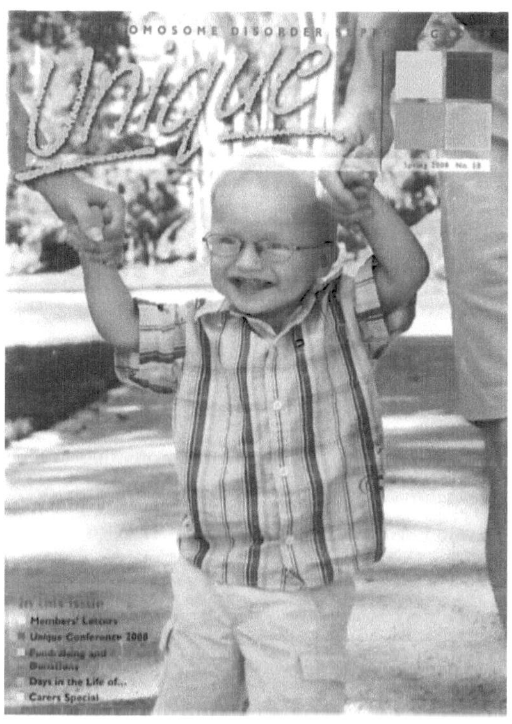

Luke on the cover of Unique *magazine*

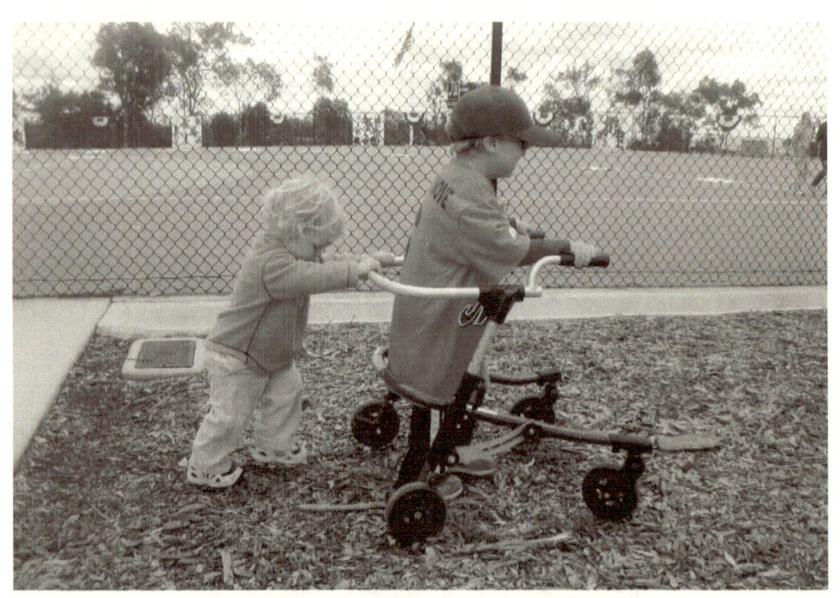

Everett, always the helper

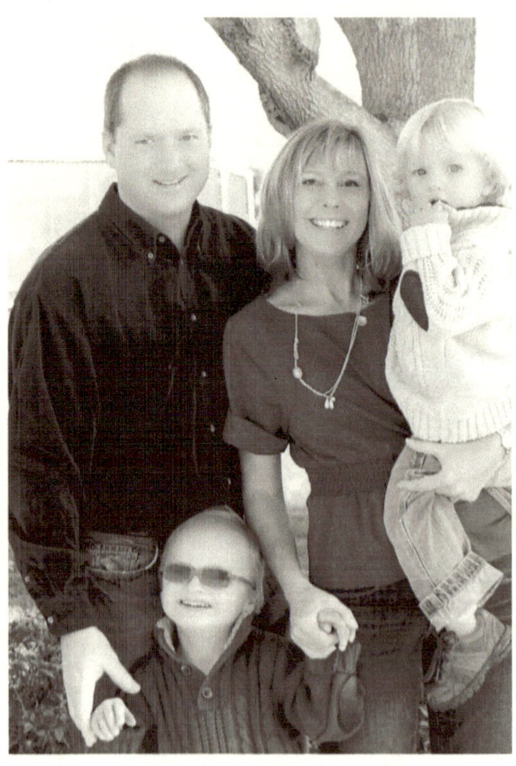

Family of 4

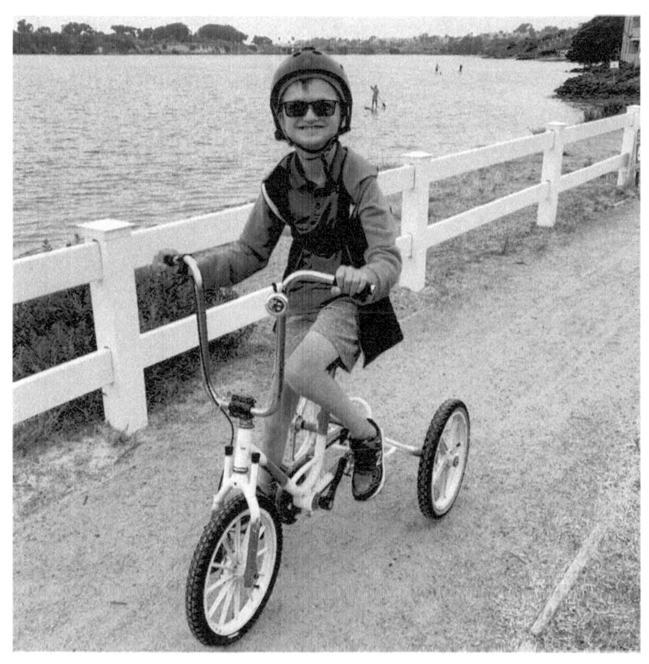

Luke riding during his "100 Mile Challenge" in June 2020

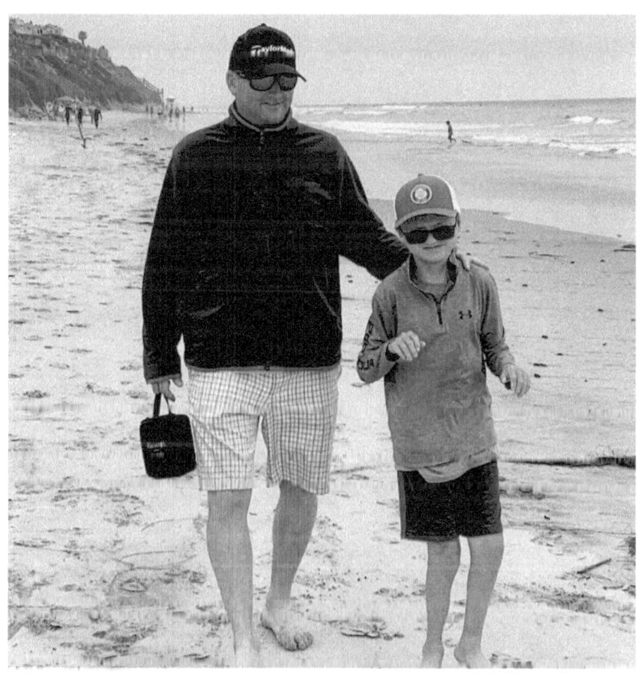

A Carlsbad beach walk with dad

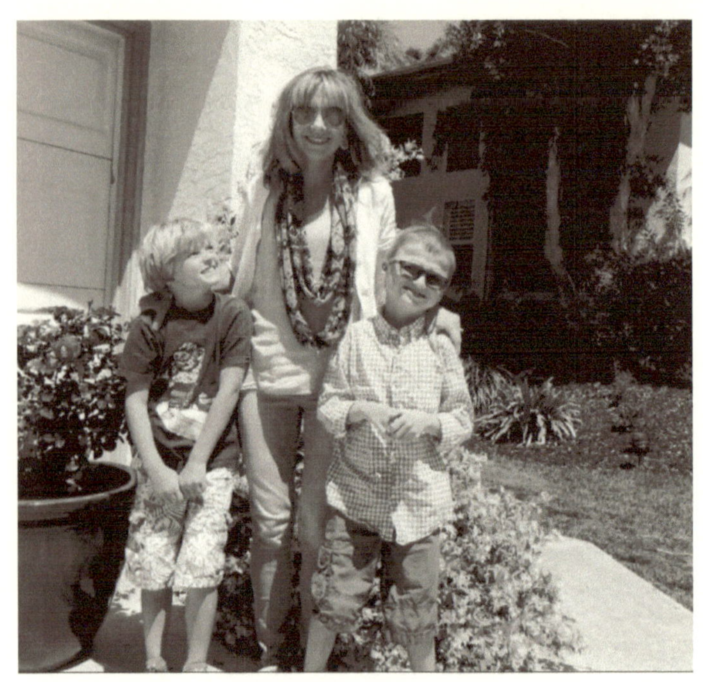

Mom and her boys

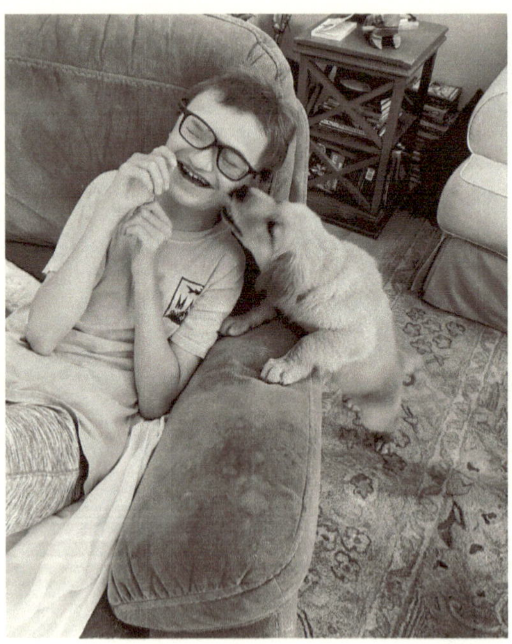

Luke with Wink, our new golden retriever puppy

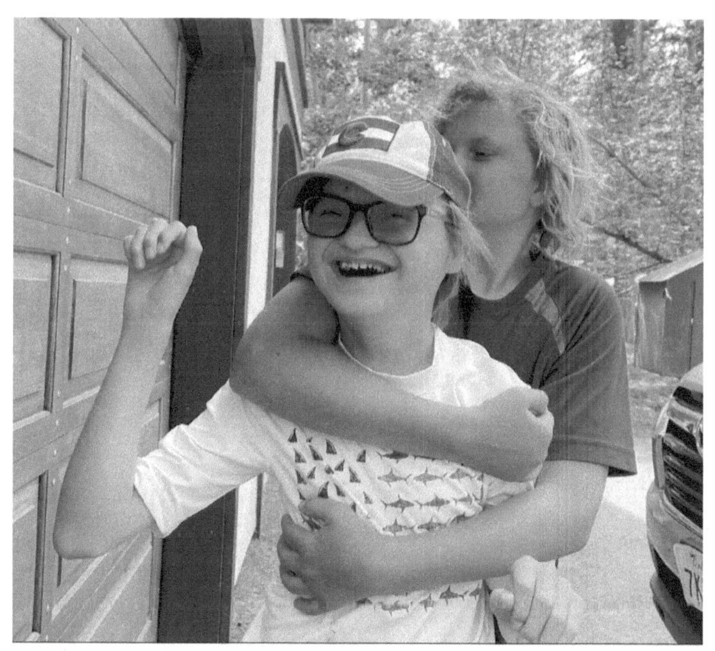

Brothers goofing around in Lake Tahoe, 2021

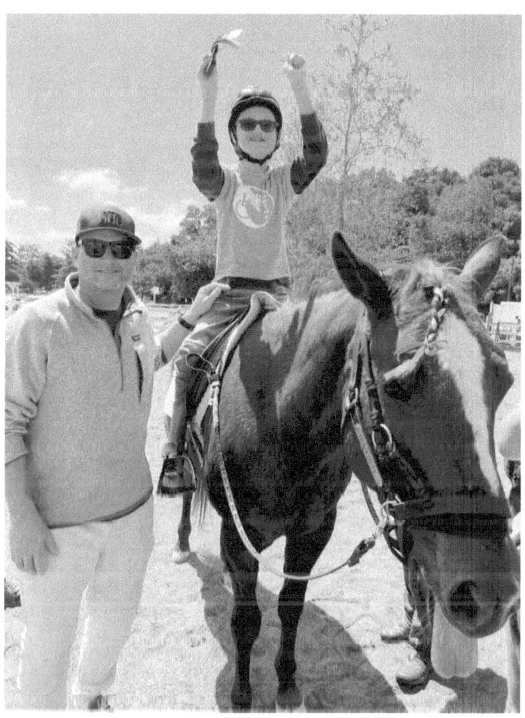

Luke at REINS for therapeutic horseback riding

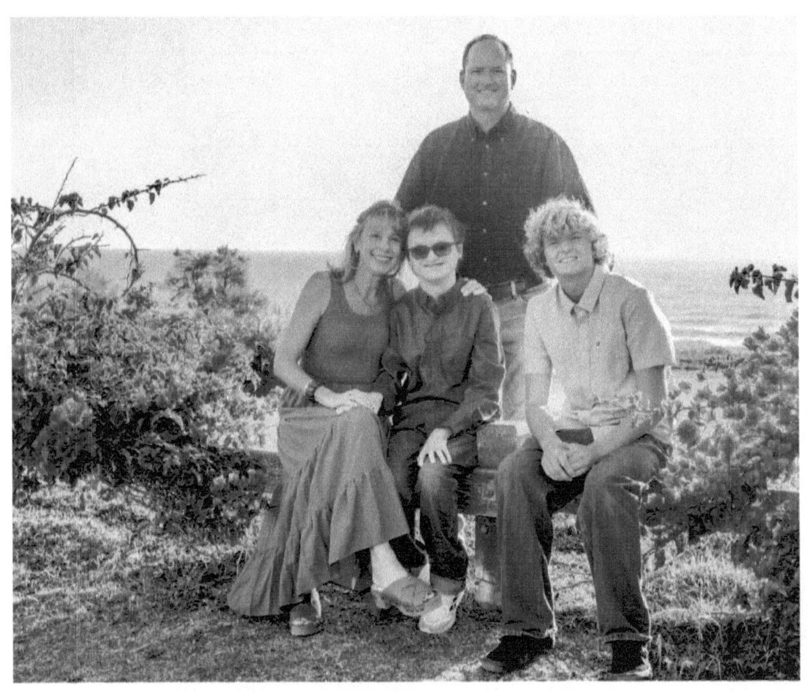

Family photo in Carlsbad, 2024

eight

Wheelchairs & the Room that Kept on Giving

I WORKED AS AN ADVOCATE FOR MANY years before taking a pause for Luke's surgery in the fall of 2018, which is also when my mom got really sick.

When Luke started middle school, we began to notice subtle changes in the way he walked. He was slightly hunched over, his feet turned inward more than ever, and his calves and hamstrings seemed unusually tight. For the first time, Luke looked genuinely uncomfortable. He has an incredibly high tolerance for pain, but this didn't seem like pain. It was more of a deep, lingering discomfort—at least, for the time being.

We knew it was time to see a doctor. We met with two orthopedic surgeons. One at Rady Children's Hospital, our home away from home, and one in a private practice. Both doctors agreed surgery would most likely be necessary, but trying medication and a few Botox treatments was a good first step. Luke's issues were most likely neurological in nature and caused his muscles to be abnormally tight and his feet to rotate inward.

Just to clarify, Botox was for Luke's tendons, not my deep creases. Though at this point, both probably could have used some attention.

We opted for the surgeon at Rady Children's Hospital. From our very first meeting, it was clear that this doctor would work well with our family. Her personality is a combination of professionalism supported by calm and kind tones and just the right touch of humor that puts everyone at ease. But what really set her apart, and honestly what sealed the deal for us, was how she interacted with Luke.

She talked to Luke. Directly to Luke. She would look him straight in the eyes and include him in our conversations. She explained medical information in a way he might be able to understand, and she treated him like the person he is, rather than just a patient file or a condition to be managed.

This might sound like basic human decency, but unfortunately, we've found it to be remarkably rare in the medical world. Too often, doctors will direct all their comments and questions to the parent or caregiver, especially when there is an intellectual disability, essentially talking over or around the patient. Luke has experienced this, and I believe that each instance chips away at his sense of dignity. Her approach was refreshing, and she recognized that Luke deserved to be an active participant in his own care.

So, we tried Baclofen, which is a medication that can reduce high tone or tightness. That was... short-lived. The doctor mentioned there could be side effects, and I vaguely recall her saying something about possible agitation. I didn't think much of it at the time.

Then, he started taking it.

Oh. My. The temper. Luke turned into an angry little gremlin. What happened to my sweet, mellow kid? I remember thinking, *Nope. Hard pass. We'll take the tight tendons over raging teen, thank you very much.* Especially since we hadn't noticed any real improvement.

The Botox route was more straightforward. The goal is for the Botox to block the nerve signals that tell the muscles to contract. We ended up doing maybe four rounds. I'd take him to the rehab doctor's office, he'd lie on the table, and I'd basically serve as a human straitjacket, lying across him while they injected the Botox into his tendons.

Just to clarify, Luke wasn't reacting to the needles. He barely felt them. What he couldn't stand was lying down while strangers touched, stretched, and adjusted his body.

I was really hopeful with the Botox. I wanted it to work. I mean, inject some magic, loosen those tight muscles, skip that part of the surgery? Yes, please.

But...nope. No difference. Not even a little.

Surgery, here we come.

Luke needed surgery for two reasons, and I'll do my best to explain them without completely butchering the medical terminology.

First, his hamstring and calf muscles had become extremely tight over time. Essentially, he has really high muscle tone, and this tone issue stems from his brain. His tendons lose their flexibility and start causing problems. The doctor planned to cut into the protective sheath surrounding those tendons, which would allow them to lengthen naturally. This procedure, combined with extensive physical therapy afterward, should give Luke significantly better range of motion, improve his overall mobility, and reduce any discomfort he's been experiencing. Essentially, we're trying to give his muscles the freedom to function properly again.

The second surgery was called guided growth surgery, and timing was crucial here. This procedure only works when someone still has growing left to do, so we couldn't wait much longer. The surgeon would insert rods and screws into both of Luke's knees and ankles, strategic hardware designed to guide his legs to grow straight during his next growth spurt. It's a bit like having internal braces that work with his body's natural growth process to correct alignment issues.

I'm fairly certain that our surgeon would have more than a few corrections to make to my oversimplified explanation, but that covers the essential points: release the tight muscles to improve function and add guidance systems to ensure proper growth alignment. Both surgeries were designed to work together to give Luke the best possible outcome for his mobility and comfort going forward.

The surgeon told me he would have casts on both legs, and I nodded along, like I was following a recipe for chocolate chip cookies. You know, simple enough… just follow the steps and hope for the best.

Apparently, I didn't ask the right questions about those casts. Because I nearly hit the floor when Luke came out of surgery looking like he'd been dipped in plaster from groin to toe. Both legs. Fully encased. No wiggle room. No knees. Just two fully cast legs, one green and one blue because that is what Luke chose, with his cute little toes popping out on the end.

I stared, blinking, trying to find words.

"How is he going to walk? No, how is he going to move?" I finally mustered up the courage to ask, still clinging to my delusions of mobility.

"Oh, he's not. Not for a while anyway."

I guess I thought the wheelchair would be optional. Or at least very temporary. Why hadn't I asked more about the casts? Why did I think we were going to somehow breeze through this like we were picking up groceries? And the practical question that hit me like a freight train: How am I ever going to keep him clean?

There was too much to think about, so I did what any reasonable person would do: I just kept putting one foot in front of the other, while Luke couldn't put either foot anywhere.

We spent one night at the hospital. Luke was on pain medication, so he was relatively comfortable and resting well. I, on the other hand, didn't sleep a wink. Every time his monitoring equipment would beep—which seemed to happen constantly—and a nurse would come in to check on him, I found myself holding my breath. I worried that even the slightest movement or the gentlest touch might cause him pain or disturb his fragile state.

Looking at him lying there, I thought of the albino koala bear. Precious and rare, needing extra care and protection. That night, watching Luke in his hospital bed, I was reminded again that Luke too was small, defenseless, and completely dependent on the people around him to keep him safe.

All I could do that night was sit in that uncomfortable hospital chair, watch over him, and pray that everything would be okay.

The first challenge in our post-surgery adventure was one that, in all my pre-operative worrying, had never even crossed my mind. How exactly do you get a kid with completely straight, immobilized legs into an SUV while still managing to buckle his seatbelt?

Fortunately, this wasn't the hospital staff's first rodeo with this type of surgery. They took one look at my slightly panicked expression and calmly told me to go get the car, drive it around to the front entrance, and a couple of them would meet me there with Luke in tow to help with what was about to become a very strategic loading operation.

Picture this automotive puzzle: three rows of seats, and we needed to figure out the perfect configuration. Luke would go in the second row on the passenger side. The front passenger seat had to be pushed as far forward as humanly possible, practically touching the dashboard. Luke's seat, meanwhile, needed to be pushed back as far as it would go. The goal was to create enough room for his legs to remain completely straight, which was non-negotiable, given his current hardware situation.

But here's where it got really tricky: getting him positioned in there. We had to move him slowly and carefully because Luke had just had hardware inserted into both his knees and ankles, plus multiple tendons had been cut. One wrong move, one slight bump or twist, and we'd be dealing with a very uncomfortable kid and possibly undoing some of the surgeon's careful work.

It was like trying to load a very precious, very fragile piece of furniture that also happened to be your son.

We did it. Got him home safely and, somehow, with Glenn's help, we got him out of the car and into our house.

We knew Luke would be setting up camp at home, or *we* would be setting up camp for Luke, for the next couple of months. So, we moved his mattress to a downstairs room that was currently being used as a playroom. It wouldn't serve that purpose anymore. It would now be Luke's space to heal—and mine, too. A place where I'd spend the next few months sleeping beside him.

The first night home, as we were getting ready to turn in—or at least pretend to turn in, or maybe just shut the lights off since Luke's sleep schedule had gone completely sideways—in walked Everett, nine years old at the time. Pillow and blanket in hand, he asked me to scoot over. He was sleeping next to me on what was maybe a full-size futon, which, trust me, was never really meant for sleeping.

Still, I scooted over. And I thought to myself, very sweet that he wants to spend the first night with us down here. Let's see if he makes it through the night.

But there he slept, not just for the night, but for the entire seven weeks that we spent in that room together.

It took seven weeks before Luke could walk up the stairs, you ask? No, he wasn't anywhere near that. But there was someone else who needed this room now. Even more than Luke.

This room was about to be transitioned once again, this time to become my beautiful mother's final resting place.

My mom. Marilyn. Grammy. She was family. She was love. She was the best cook and baker I knew. She was beautiful, inside and out. And in her own way, she was fragile.

She lived in Carlsbad part-time and spent quality time with all of us. She made these amazing Sunday night dinners that always had no less than two entrees, an array of side dishes, and at least three dessert options. Did I mention she was under 100 pounds? A petite woman who had the gift of being able to produce the most amazing baked goods without overindulging herself. A trait that I did not inherit.

She truly had a heart of gold.

Now, she was close to entering hospice. She had been diagnosed with Stage 4 lung cancer almost two years prior. Our 65-year-old, non-smoking, healthy, professional-grade cook and baker suddenly had lung cancer that had spread to her brain and spinal fluid. The diagnosis felt impossible. How does someone who never smoked, who took care of herself, end up with lung cancer?

She was treated at Northwestern, near her part-time home in the Chicago area, and for a brief, hopeful period, we thought she might beat the odds. The doctors were cautiously optimistic, and we allowed ourselves to believe that maybe, just maybe, she would be one of the lucky few. But even after every intervention—targeted radiation, chemotherapy, immunotherapy, surgery, all the latest experimental medications—nothing could prevent the cancer from continuing its relentless march through her body.

After months of her resisting our suggestions and fiercely wanting to maintain her independence, there came a point where we all recognized that she should be closer to family. It made perfect sense for her to move back to Carlsbad, a place she knew and loved, and where she had so many happy memories. Plus, practically speaking, we had a bedroom and full bathroom on the first floor, the same room where Luke had been recovering.

Now, we just had to relocate Luke, casts and all, ready or not, back upstairs to his bedroom. The timing wasn't ideal, but then again, nothing about this situation was ideal.

We were nearing the end, and we needed her to be with us. She needed us, too, but what I knew for sure was that I needed my mom. I needed her close. I needed her safe.

This is what happens when you're navigating the complicated world of special needs parenting: real life doesn't pause for your crisis. It just keeps layering on, one challenge at a time, until you're managing recovery from major surgery while preparing to say goodbye to the person who taught you how to be strong in the first place.

After 4 ½ months with us, my mom passed away on May 12th, 2019. It was Mother's Day.

I think back to those months, and there were some almost impossible days. Anyone who has cared for a loved one until the end understands what I mean. You find yourself pushing aside grief so you can put on even the slightest semblance of hope, not just for them but for yourself. Because without that tiny thread of hope, you might not make it through the day.

I felt a constant, heavy tiredness deep in my bones. There was fear, sharp and relentless, the kind that tightens your chest when you think about what tomorrow might bring. There was sadness, sometimes so overwhelming it made even small tasks feel impossible. And there was that quiet, gnawing grief that hovered in the background, refusing to be ignored.

Yet, through it all, there was fierce, unyielding, and raw love. A love that made every sleepless night, every anxious moment, every heartbreak worth it, even as it broke me open. I was scared and hopeful, grieving and grateful, terrified and stubbornly resilient, all at once.

My mom, who had always been adamant that she would never take opioids or even more than one or two over-the-counter pain meds during the day, became someone I was constantly trying to coax into taking pain medication. I'd try to slip pills into her food, sometimes into her tea, with little to no success. She had this uncanny ability to know exactly what I was up to, no matter how sneaky I thought I was being.

Then came the 2 AM screams of pain—those gut-wrenching moments when she'd tell me her pain was a 12 out of 10, and I'd finally convince her to take the pain medication. She'd take it, find some relief, and then forget it all the next morning, repeating that same cycle each day.

You see, the tumors had spread to her brain, which affected her memory. But the tumors had also spread to her spinal fluid, something that was first noticed in a test while she was still at Northwestern.

The oncologist described the cancer there as if the tumors were like crystallized sugar, floating through her spinal fluid. There wasn't much they could do to treat that except try new medications that might buy more time, but those came with some pretty harsh side effects.

And those little crystallized tumors? They caused excruciating pain. They also caused double vision, which was heartbreaking to watch. Here was this woman who had always been so sharp, so aware, struggling to see clearly and remember from one day to the next.

We had caregivers—two exceptional women, Bonnie and Ann—who were there through it all, and I still call them friends today. They helped make what felt unmanageable somehow manageable.

Because through all of this, we still had to take care of Luke. And Luke still needed a lot of care. Glenn and I carried him up and down the stairs each day for months. He absolutely refused to bend his knees, despite his surgeon and his physical therapist telling us there was no physical reason for this.

He was simply terrified to bend his knees.

Scary Barry

Once Luke's casts were off, we did months of physical therapy a couple times a week, not too far from our home, in a building that looked like a castle, with a physical therapist we will call Barry. It became quite the tradition. Afternoon PT appointments followed by some good food because nothing says, "We survived another session," quite like comfort eating.

Barry was a genuinely nice man with years of experience working with children. We felt confident in our decision to work with him to get Luke walking again. We were starting with a more realistic goal: the slightest bend of his legs. Baby steps, literally.

There was absolutely nothing scary about Barry. He was patient, kind, and had that gentle demeanor you want in someone working with kids. The only terrifying thing about him was the simple fact that he was the person working with Luke to get his legs moving again.

Luke absolutely hated going to see Barry. And honestly, who could blame him? His legs had been slashed open, hardware had been inserted, he'd endured months of casts, and somehow the surgery had left him with the most sensitive toes known to mankind. I don't know what happened during that procedure, but afterward, I couldn't even accidentally brush against Luke's toes without him twisting his entire body and making the most uncomfortable noises I've ever heard.

So, naturally, he did not want anyone messing with him or his legs. He also deeply resented every minute of walking practice or attempting to walk up and down stairs as part of his therapy. In Luke's mind, Barry wasn't helping him get better; Barry was the guy who made him do hard, uncomfortable things twice a week.

It didn't matter that we explained to Luke why he had to do physical therapy or that Barry was gentle and encouraging. To Luke, physical therapy was torture, and Barry was the friendly face of that torture.

Over time, all the therapy worked. Luke mustered up the courage to finally bend his knees one day in our backyard while riding his adult, modified trike. We had been carefully lifting him and placing him on his trike, hoping he would want to ride and that the motivation would help bend his knees. Then, one day, for a brief moment, I think he forgot about his self-imposed knee-bending boycott, and he just started pedaling like a typical kid.

The moment he realized what he was doing, he panicked and stopped mid-pedal, probably thinking, *Wait, what am I doing? I'm supposed to hate this!* He looked over at us, and there we were, Glenn and I, cheering for him like he had just won the Tour de France.

Luke smiled his beautiful smile and kept riding, finally remembering that using his knees was actually kind of fun.

So, yes. Thank you, Barry, for all of those "horrible" sessions that

Luke absolutely despised. Thank you for being patient with a kid who acted like you were personally responsible for every uncomfortable moment in his life. Thank you for not taking it personally when Luke looked at you like you were the villain.

Turns out, all that torture disguised as physical therapy worked.

My plan was to go back to advocacy in early 2020, but remember what happened then? The pandemic. You know, that global event that turned everyone's life upside down and inside out. Suddenly, like parents everywhere, the boys were home full time, and we quickly transitioned to online school—which, let me tell you, was about as smooth as you'd expect with anything involving technology.

In many ways, we were fortunate, and I mean that sincerely. Glenn and I were both home with the boys. He worked from home during the days, while I became the unofficial homeschool coordinator, IT support, snack distributor, and referee all rolled into one. We went on countless neighborhood walks because we HAD to get out of the house each day or risk completely losing our minds. I'm pretty sure our neighbors thought we were training for a marathon based on how often they saw us circling the block.

We also had Luke's instructional aide from school with us who worked for an agency but was provided by our school district five mornings a week. That's right; our school district sent a qualified aide to our home to work with Luke. We are in a pretty amazing district with a director who put students before budget during this trying time. She was on virtual school calls with him, working on goals and life skills. She even ate lunch with Luke, Everett, and me. She became part of our bubble. It was a lifesaver, or at least a sanity saver, for me, and a bonding experience for both boys.

We quickly settled into a routine that felt both comforting and completely surreal: morning exercise because movement helps with focus, a good breakfast, a little schoolwork that may or may not have qualified as actual learning, maybe an afternoon movie or the latest

Netflix series, then a bit more schoolwork. We planned the next week's meals because suddenly life revolved around what we were going to cook and eat together, waited for the weekly grocery delivery, and ended the day with a meal we had time to savor together.

Food became our obsession. Like, we were seriously obsessed. We were making everything from scratch: bread, pasta, elaborate desserts that required ingredients we'd never heard of. Family dinners became these epic productions where we'd spend hours cooking together and then sit around the table, talking to each other without anyone checking their phone. I have these photos of the delicious, creative food we made together, and I often wish I had the time and energy to keep it all up today. But for now, it's back to a lot of semi-homemade food and dinner together a few days a week if we're lucky.

But I digress. No outside work for me during the pandemic. I took some phone calls and talked with parents who had children in special education about making the most of this time, but I had no meetings or much advocacy work for now. We lived in our little bubble, stayed healthy, binge-watched so many series, and enjoyed this forced family time. One of the coolest things Luke and I did during the pandemic was his June 100-mile challenge with Ainsley's Angels, an organization that offers all-inclusive endurance events in our communities. They pair athletes and runners with people with disabilities who could not otherwise compete in endurance events. In-person races were canceled, so even Ainsley's Angels went virtual. Luke rode his trike, with me by his side, 100 miles in June 2020. All around our neighborhood, Mission Bay, Coronado—all over San Diego. He loved it, and wow, did we sleep well that month!

In March 2021, knowing that the boys would be returning to school in the foreseeable future, I made the decision to start advocating again.

Shannon had sold PCA to one of our former colleagues, who was also a parent advocate, and I considered returning and working for her. It would have been the safe choice, but after years of experience and way too much time to think during lockdown, I decided that it was time to start my own business. Apparently, I'm a glutton for punishment, and the stress of working for someone else wasn't quite enough. I needed the added anxiety of being responsible for everything myself.

I dabbled in t-shirt making during the pandemic—optimism t-shirts, to be exact, because if there was ever a time the world needed more optimism, it was 2020. I had some fun with it until my heat press broke (of course, it did), and any new design ideas involved cursing or wine references, which seemed inappropriate for a family business. That business was named Blue Glasses Co. because Luke has always worn, and I guess now always will wear, blue glasses, so it seemed personal and appropriate. Plus, it was one of the few business names that wasn't already taken by someone else, which felt like a small miracle.

I decided to keep going with that concept because I really wasn't in the mood to overthink anything anymore, so I started Blue Glasses Advocacy. No business plan, no market research, just me, my laptop, and my years of experience.

I wrote up a contract (thank goodness for templates), a release of information, set up email accounts, and created a website that was basically a few pages of, "Here's who I am, and here's how I can help." That made me feel official. I registered as a sole proprietorship, got my business license, paid my fees, and boom! I was in business. It felt both terrifying and exhilarating.

I remember my first client like it was yesterday: a concerned and caring family with a kindergartener who wasn't getting the services he needed. No, I didn't mention to the parents that they were my very first "on my own" client. I was nervous enough jumping back into the advocacy game, let alone doing it by myself for the first time. They didn't need to know they were my guinea pigs. I must have spent three times longer than necessary preparing for that first IEP meeting, researching every possible scenario, every regulation, and every potential argument. I was determined not to screw it up.

It went great. The child got appropriate services, the parents were relieved, and I realized I may actually be able to pull this off.

I got busier quicker than I thought I would, which was both amazing and slightly panic-inducing. Referrals from other advocates and special education attorneys started coming my way, and I never had to place the ads I'd crafted because word of mouth in the special education world travels fast. When you do good work, people talk. When you mess up, they talk even faster.

It was pretty part-time at first, squeezed in between school pickups and surf team practices, but through the years, it has become darn close to a full-time job—but one with flexibility. And now that the boys are older, it's one I can find balance with, most days. It still has me searching special education regulations because, apparently, even after all these years, I'm still far from having all the answers. The learning curve never ends; it just gets more interesting.

I still love what I do. Like, genuinely love it in a way that surprises me sometimes. I am still getting out of my comfort zone every single day and walking into rooms with people who've been doing this longer than I have, although as time goes on, the IEP teams keep getting younger and younger. I'm advocating for kids whose situations are more complex than anything I learned about in training and having conversations with parents who are at their absolute breaking point and trusting me to help them navigate the system.

I continue to meet and work with some of the most amazing families—parents who would move mountains for their kids, siblings who become fierce advocates themselves, and grandparents who show up to every meeting, armed with questions and determination. These families remind me daily why this work matters.

And I am still learning every day, which I believe continues to help both of my boys with their education. Luke still needs an advocate, and he just happens to live with one. Everett has learned more about student rights and self-advocacy than most adults understand, just from hearing me talk about my work and seeing how we handle challenges in our own family.

Is it easy? No way. Some weeks, I feel like I'm on fire at IEP meetings. And then, there are the days when I'm eating cereal for dinner and again wondering if I've completely lost my mind trying to build a business while raising kids. But it is meaningful work, and managing my own schedule and choosing exactly how busy I want to be gives me a balance that makes it all possible.

Love Lesson from a Mom

Sometimes, love doesn't look like hugs and comfort. Sometimes love looks like insisting on the hard things, the things our kids would rather avoid, things that make them uncomfortable, even things that make them a little mad at us in the moment.

As a mom, it broke my heart to see Luke glare at Barry like he was the enemy. I wanted to scoop him up, protect him from the struggle, and whisper, "You don't have to do this if you don't want to." But I knew that letting him skip the hard stuff—therapy, exercises, the repetitive motions that make muscles stretch and grow—would have been stealing from his future. Love is letting someone dislike you a little in the moment, while you stand firm for their tomorrow. It's trusting that the frustration, the tears, and even the resentment won't last, but that the lessons, the strength, and the progress will. It's showing up over and over, even when the path is messy and the victories are tiny. It's understanding that the hard things are where courage grows, resilience is built, and independence begins to take shape.

Love is sitting beside them when they push back, quietly holding the line, even when your heart aches with every grimace, every protest, every refusal. It's celebrating the small wins and knowing that these moments, so easily overlooked, are the building blocks of confidence, self-reliance, and strength.

Love is letting go, just enough to let them stumble, to let them try, to let them feel the discomfort that teaches them they are capable. It's remembering that every tear, every groan, every glare in the moment is a sign of growth in disguise. And when the day comes that they finally succeed, when they meet the challenge on their own, the joy is multiplied because it was earned through patience, persistence, and faith.

Sometimes love means getting up in the middle of the night, wiping tears, and whispering words of comfort even when there are no right words. Love is being present and saying, *"I won't let you face this alone."*

Love is messy, demanding, sometimes invisible, and yet even with all its hard edges, it is also the most powerful teacher of all.

Luke's smile that day on the trike when he finally bent his knees was my reminder.

nine

WE'RE NOT **THAT** FAMILY...
OH, YES, WE ARE

ONE MORNING LUKE HAD AN EARLY DENTIST appointment, and since he barely tolerated those visits and the straitjacket—I mean "papoose"—that had to be used to get a decent cleaning, I decided to let him play hooky from school that afternoon. When we got home from the dentist, Luke asked to ride his trike. Perfect idea. Exercise for him, and I could water the plants. He circled happily in our U-shaped backyard while I grabbed the hose. Since we live in California, where most lawns are tiny and drought rules are strict, I figured I'd take two minutes to water the front as well. I double-locked the gate to the yard, confident Luke was safe. Every inch of our house had been professionally babyproofed.

But when I came back, the gate stood wide open.

What? I didn't leave it open. Did I? Was I finally losing it? Sleep-deprived dementia setting in? My stomach dropped. I sprinted around the yard—no Luke. Checked the kitchen—empty. I looked up at the hillside (ridiculous, but I checked anyway). His trike was gone, too.

He had figured out the locks. Both of them. For the very first time.

Shit.

Luke was gone.

I went into full panic mode. I ran to the front, but there was no sign of him. I grabbed my keys and tore off, barefoot, in the car. Luke could have taken the cul-de-sac loop safely enough. Or he could have gone up the hill, still manageable. But if he turned right? That road. Six lanes. Fifty-five miles per hour. My heart stopped. I headed there first.

I drove like a crazy woman. No full stops. No regard for traffic lights. Just terror. I combed the road, did a U-turn, and checked again. Nothing. Relief mixed with dread.

I turned up the hill. As I crawled past a side path near our house, I spotted him. Luke was still strapped into his trike, helmet on, wedged in a bush. Not upright, not quite safe, but alive. His eyes were wide, scared, waiting. I ran, unbuckled him, and pulled him close. I don't think I had ever held him that tightly.

"Luke, you're safe," I whispered into his hair.

Lesson learned, the hard way: all that occupational therapy had paid off. He could now undo locks. And I would never, ever leave him unattended again. Not even a few yards away. Not even for two minutes.

To any of my neighbors who saw me driving barefoot, hair wild, yelling into the street like a madwoman, now you know why.

I am that mom. We are that family.

Travel Diaries

Luke was a great traveler when he was young. And by "great," I mean he tolerated long TSA lines, airport chaos, and hours-long flights without having a complete meltdown. And by "young," I mean under the age of four, before life, anxiety, and sensory overload decided to join us for the ride.

Our family is scattered all over the country, so in those early years, we made the rounds with Luke in tow. Chicago, Minneapolis, Nashville, Florida, Arizona, and LA.

He even handled London and Paris like a little jet-setter just before his third birthday. We were bracing ourselves for the 12-hour flight, fully prepared for meltdown central, but Luke was a champ.

In fact, when we landed, the man sitting directly behind us tapped us on the shoulder. He said, "I'll be honest, when you sat down with that little guy, I thought, 'Here we go.' But your kid? He either slept or smiled the whole way." Luke had his adorable blue glasses perched on his oversized toddler head—picture Chicken Little meets the kid from *Jerry Maguire*. And when he wasn't sleeping, he was smiling at everyone. All. Flight. Long.

We made many trips to see family in those early years—visits with my side of the family in Chicago and Minneapolis, and with Glenn's family in Florida and Nashville. During one trip, we arrived late in the evening, and Glenn's mom, Joan, had thoughtfully put out a bedside rail so Luke could sleep without falling out of the bed.

We put him down, and he screamed. And cried. And thirty minutes later, he was still crying. So much for sleep anytime soon. It was clear this bed idea was a no-go.

So Glenn and his dad did what any desperate, sleep-deprived person would do: they ran to Walmart at 11:45 PM (it closed at midnight), raced through the store, and grabbed the very last pack-n-play. They brought it back, set it up, and finally, Luke slept.

Every time I think of Walmart, I can't help but remember that night. The stress, the chaos, and the lengths we went to just to get a little rest. And somehow, even in the middle of all that madness, it's one of our favorite Luke stories.

We had our parental worries back then—of course, we did. But travel-related behavior wasn't one of them.

And then, something shifted.

I can't tell you exactly when it happened. Whether it crept in slowly or showed up overnight like an uninvited guest, but somewhere along the way, something changed.

Let's call it anxiety.

Crowds? Overstimulating. Noise? Overwhelming. Being out in public with us, Mom and Dad? Apparently, that's a trigger.

Here's the kicker: his behaviors only seem to escalate when he's with us. His parents. You know, the people who provide unconditional love and snacks on demand. His so-called "safe place." Ironically, that seems to be the very thing that flips the switch.

And according to many, this isn't uncommon. "Kids act out most around their parents because they feel safest with them." Sure, okay, fine. But I'm still not 100% sold. Luke's school team? They're incredible. They're his people. His safe place, too. So, why is it so different with us?

Is it hormones? Is it trauma? Is it that he knows we'll love him no matter what, and so he lets it all out when he's near us?

I don't have the answer. But what I do know is that we are THAT family.

We Still Travel, But Let's Be Real About It

I'll start with not one, but two of our favorite travel bloopers.

We were back in Florida to visit Glenn's parents when Luke was around 10 or 11 years old. No more pack-n-play—we had bigger issues to deal with. We try to keep Luke's morning routine as close to home as possible, so one early morning, he was sitting on the toilet with his iPad in hand. Normally, this routine goes off without a hitch, but that morning, his iPad lost its connection. Frustrated, Luke didn't stand up and ask for help. No. He decided to have some fun with one of his favorite pastimes: flushing the toilet. Only this time, he spiced things up by flushing his pajama bottoms down it. Before we knew it, water was rushing out of the bathroom. Glenn turned off the water, the plumber arrived, fished the pajamas out, and handed us a hefty bill.

Fast forward five years. We're back in Florida again, and Luke is back on the toilet. Like the responsible parents we think we are, we remembered the pajama bottom story, so off those went, and we even cleared the entire bathroom counter. All was calm—or so we thought. The iPad was working fine this time, but Luke has an exceptionally good memory. Somehow, he opened a drawer, found a washcloth, and, yes, flushed that down the toilet this time. Luke never does anything like this at home. But he remembered. Maybe it was the attention. Maybe it was the plumber. Who knows? But he remembered.

This time, when Glenn tried to turn off the water, the lever wouldn't budge. We called a neighbor who brought some sort of wrench and managed to stop the flow, but not before a bit of damage had been done. Luke was laughing, I was crying, and Glenn... well, let's just say he's the most patient person in the family, but this time there was a complete meltdown in the kitchen that involved both Luke and Glenn.

To top it all off, we were about to leave for our flight home. This was right after the pandemic, so even an emergency plumber couldn't get there for 18 hours. I kept apologizing to Mom. "We'll cover the bill. We hope we'll still be invited back."

We still travel with Luke. These days, it's mostly road trips, but we do manage to get him on an airplane once or twice a year, with a lot of planning, pre-planning, backup planning, and more planning.

We call TSA Cares ahead of time. It's a wonderful service when the airport is properly staffed and ready for us, which, in our experience, is about 50% of the time. The other half? Well, that's when we find out the "care" part is more of a suggestion than a guarantee.

We always pre-plan our airplane seating: two rows, two seats per row, one directly behind the other. Luke *must* sit behind either me or Glenn. Why? Because Luke kicks. Not sometimes. Not maybe. He kicks. And the average air traveler does *not* appreciate becoming the drum kit for a kid with strong legs and zero impulse control. I don't blame them. I wouldn't like it either. But you only need to get chewed out by one very angry passenger to learn that lesson the hard way.

We also request a wheelchair at the airport. Luke walks, so this isn't about mobility. It's about containment. With the wheelchair, we can keep him seated, give him his iPad and headphones, and make our way through the chaos of security without completely losing our minds (or our child). Even then, it's not foolproof.

Take our recent trip to Minneapolis. We had everything: TSA Cares, a wheelchair, the iPad, headphones, his favorite stuffed bear, the works. And yet, Luke still managed to smack a pregnant TSA agent.

To be clear, he didn't *mean* to hit her. His arms started flailing in sensory overload, and she just happened to be in his path. She was fine, thankfully. I, on the other hand, needed a Xanax. Why didn't I *have* Xanax?

Oh, the stares. The judgment. I knew everyone in the security line was thinking, "Thank goodness we're not that family."

Even when we go to the most beautiful places, like the North Shore of Hawaii or, most recently, Maui, the trip still comes with the same constant refrain. Every day. No, every hour. "Home soon?"

Repeated. Relentless. Sometimes, I want to scream, "NO! We're not going home soon! We're in Hawaii! We have one week! One beautiful, amazing week! I wish we weren't going home anytime soon!"

Of course, I don't say that. Not exactly. Instead, we show Luke the calendar and cross off each day so he can *see* that we're staying for now, but eventually, we will go home. Still, it doesn't stop the questions.

Restaurants while traveling? Oh, they're a whole *event*.

Like many neurodivergent people, and probably many other people in general, Luke has a very hard time regulating himself when his entire world is turned upside down—and travel flips everything. His routines are gone. His cozy bedroom is missing. Everything smells different, sounds different, and feels different. His body knows it. His brain knows it. And that makes dinner with linen napkins and glassware... risky.

On a recent birthday dinner for Everett, we cleared the table—bare minimum silverware, no extra plates, and zero butter knives in sight. And yet, Luke still managed to find a glass and… crash. Mood instantly gone. The birthday boy sighed. I cried. We really tried. But yeah, it's easier to barbecue by the pool. More space. Less breakables.

We are not a hotel family. We rent condos or houses with full kitchens and actual bedrooms. Sounds nice, right? "Oooh, you and Glenn get your own bedroom!"

Ha. No.

Luke travels with an REI camping mattress and sleeps on the floor, directly next to our bed. It's the only way I sleep. Rentals may be better than hotels, but they are still not Luke-proof.

And by Luke-proof, I mean as soon as I walk into a rental, I'm scanning like a secret service agent. I have already studied the online listing's floor plan before we even left home, weeks in advance.

When we arrive, it's "go time."

Kitchen first. Knife block? Put that beast on top of the fridge. Every drawer gets checked for sharp objects just waiting to be discovered.

Bedrooms next. We don't always use the "primary bedroom." We pick the one with the safest layout. I pad the sides of Luke's mattress, stuff pillows under the bed so he doesn't roll under, unplug lamps and remove them along with the side tables, move artwork, wrap cords from the blinds, and hide every vase or knick-knack like Luke's life depends on it. And it just might.

I take photos of everything before moving it, so we can put the house back together before we check out, like a responsible, neurotic criminal. I mean, guest.

And no leather furniture. Ever. Once, Luke sat on my dad's very expensive leather chair and dragged his fingernails across both armrests while watching his iPad. The scratches? Permanent. The damage? Done. Thankfully, my dad was cool about it. Still, no leather. Ever again.

We also bring pads. Lots of them. For chairs, couches, mattresses.

The kind meant to protect against leaks. You know the kind. You do what you gotta do.

I'm proud to say that I have many 5-star rental reviews, and I've earned every single one of them.

Traveling is exhausting. Keeping Luke safe while traveling is exhausting. Sleeping while traveling is... mostly theoretical.

But we keep doing it.

Not because it's easy. Not because it's "worth it" in the Instagram sense.

But because our family still deserves to go places. Even when it's hard. Especially when it's hard.

Because this is what traveling looks like for us, and we are THAT family.

Oh, yes, we are.

We Are Also THAT Family, Right Here at Home

It's not just at the airport. Or in rentals. Or on some dream vacation we paid too much for and barely remember because we were running on fumes.

Nope. We are also THAT family right here at home. Neighborhood restaurants. Grocery store runs. Even backyard barbecues. No place is completely safe.

My first vivid memory of Luke acting out in public? He was five. We were visiting Glenn's brother, John, in L.A., which is just over an hour north of us, and we had just wrapped up a beautiful, overstimulating, sun-soaked day at the Santa Monica Pier. Naturally, I thought, *Let's end the day with a nice meal. Let's go to Duke's in Malibu!*

Risky? Oh, yes. Worth it? We thought so. It was Duke's. Ocean views, fresh fish, tropical drinks—how bad could it be?

At first, it was everything we hoped for: the view was breathtaking, the food and drink were top-tier, and the server? Kind, welcoming, and accommodating.

We were chatting with him, placing our order, sipping drinks, soaking it all in...

And then, out of nowhere, *CRACK!* Luke picked up a salad plate and hurled it at the server's head. Like with intent. A clean, fast, overhand toss. Narrowly missed.

The whole table froze. *Did that just...? Did Luke...?*

No. It couldn't be Luke. Not our sweet, smiling Luke. The boy with the baby face and blue glasses? The one who looked like a Pixar character and had people smiling at him wherever he went.

Yup. It was him. No mistake. Plate tossed. Server nearly concussed.

Maybe we didn't include him in the conversation. Maybe he was hungry. Maybe he got a weird vibe from our server and trusted his instincts. (Was he right? We'll never know.)

All I knew in that moment was that Luke was mad, and he wanted that server gone. Immediately.

I was mortified. The apologies began. To the server's credit, he took a breath, smiled (a little tighter this time), and said, "It's okay. I'll be back soon with your food."

The rest of the dinner, believe it or not, went off without a hitch. But that moment? That was the beginning of our very long, very dramatic, ongoing relationship with restaurants. That's the day the restaurant rules were born.

We have a system now.

Rule #1: Table scouting. Just like I scope out vacation rentals online weeks in advance, I now walk into restaurants like an interior designer/strategic operations commander. Not every table works. In fact, most tables do not work. The table must be as far away as possible from other diners, next to a window for a distraction (I mean view), and in the corner, if possible, as we find much success tucking Luke into the corner pocket.

Yes. We put baby in a corner.

(*Cue Patrick Swayze voice*: "Nobody puts Baby in a corner."

Actually, Patrick, we absolutely do. It's for everyone's safety.)

Rule #2: Snacks out as soon as we sit down. Eating while ordering ensures a better outcome every time.

Rule #3: No small talk with the waiter. This will never feel natural, but small talk is a trap. Stay focused. We are there to eat, not network.

Rule #4: Nothing within Luke's reach. This includes but is not limited to silverware, menus, bread baskets, pepper grinders, centerpieces, candles, ketchup bottles, laminated dessert menus, butter knives shaped like swords, water glasses, and yes, salad plates.

Rule #5: Introduce Luke immediately. Quick smile, "This is Luke," name exchange, eye contact (optional), and then we keep him involved in the (very short) ordering process so he knows he's part of it. Keep **Rule #2** in mind at all times.

Rule #6: Order Luke's food without delay. Before drinks. Before napkins. Get that food order in! Food equals a happy Luke.

Rule #7: More snacks. Always. We pack snacks like we're training for the apocalypse.

But let's be real—it's not just restaurants. This isn't just a "dining out with special needs" issue. The behaviors go way beyond dinner plates and corner booths.

Sometimes, it's at the grocery store. Sometimes, it's a meltdown on the sidewalk. Sometimes, it's during a neighborhood BBQ when he suddenly decides he needs to go home.

And if there's no salad plate to toss? Luke will find something else. A pinch. A hit. Occasionally, a bite. Not malicious, but enough to leave a mark on your arm and your soul. It's usually reserved for me and Glenn, the elite club of "People He Feels Safe Enough to Unleash On."

Though I should mention our dear friend Kerry gets the occasional pinch, too. She's known him for a long time. It's almost an honor, like we should congratulate her for making the list.

At home, our neighbors have said, "I don't know how you do it," and not in that throwaway, small-talk kind of way. I mean, they've seen it.

They've witnessed Luke knock the glasses right off my face because I dared to say hi to someone. Or slap the phone out of my hand because I made the mistake of talking to someone while he was standing next to me. Not because he's being bad. Not because he's mean. Because he's overloaded and completely overwhelmed.

And maybe I didn't include him in the conversation. And that was just too much.

Maybe I'll never fully know the "why." I try to figure it out. I *want* to figure it out. But sometimes, I just can't. And that's the part that can break you. The not knowing.

Because after all of it, after the pinch or the hit or the flying phone, Luke is just as sweet as ever. The same kid who loves his home and who melts you with a single look and doesn't even realize he's doing it.

He doesn't mean to hurt us. He's not trying to hurt us.

It comes from frustration and a lack of words. And too many feelings in a body that's still figuring out what to do with all of them.

I know this. I remind myself of it constantly.

But damn, it's hard. It's hard when your glasses are on the ground. It's hard when your arm stings and your heart does, too. It's hard when all you wanted was to wave at a neighbor and feel somewhat typical for five seconds.

I love Luke more than I will ever be able to put into words, but wow... it is really hard sometimes.

We are THAT family who skips birthday parties unless we've pre-cleared the location, menu, guest list, and noise levels.

We are THAT family who brings our own utensils, snacks, seat pads, and wipes—everywhere.

We are THAT family who leaves early, declines invitations, and has to bail last minute, not because we don't care but because our kid is already running at capacity, and we can see the crash coming before it hits.

We are THAT family who has a code word between parents to signal, "Stop talking. Stop breathing. Just stop until Luke calms down." The word is butterfly—a beautiful word for a not-so-beautiful moment.

And yes, we are THAT family who once ruined a perfectly lovely dinner at Duke's in Malibu with a rogue salad plate.

But you know what else we are? We are the family who tries anyway.

We go out. We show up. We take the risk. We mess up. We apologize. We learn. We laugh later (usually). We show our kids the world, even when the world doesn't make space for Luke.

We love big. We adapt constantly. We do the work, even when the work is really, really hard.

Because this is our life. This is Luke's life.

And we wouldn't trade it, broken salad plates and all.

We may not have planned to be that family... but we are.

Oh, yes, we are.

Love Lesson from a Mom

Love means showing up, even when it's messy. It's knowing the night might end in tears, in an early exit, or in a broken plate, but going anyway because life is worth living out loud, not hidden away.

Love is learning that joy doesn't come from perfect moments but from brave ones. From taking risks, packing extra everything, and whispering "butterfly" when it all feels like too much.

Because love isn't about making life easier. It's about making sure life is lived—fully, bravely, and unapologetically.

Love is claiming space in a world that sometimes forgets to make room. It's believing that every small victory—a shared smile, a short outing that didn't end in tears, a stranger's kindness—matters.

Love is letting your child experience the world, even when the world isn't designed for them, and gently reminding them with every outing, "You belong here, exactly as you are. You are uniquely, fully, enough."

ten

MARRIED WITH CHILDREN—
SPECIAL NEEDS EDITION

GLENN AND I MET ON AUGUST 6, 1999. We were set up on a blind date at a local restaurant known for its wide variety of beer and burgers. In other words, the ideal setting for a situation that could go either way: a heartwarming success story or an unforgettable Friday evening that should have been spent at home. The whole thing had been orchestrated by Julie, a mutual acquaintance whose matchmaking confidence far exceeded her knowledge of either of us. She was one of Glenn's clients and also the roommate of a friend of mine. I had met her exactly once before she decided to set me up. That alone probably should've been a red flag. But apparently, one meeting over margaritas gave her all the information she needed to start the matchmaking process.

There was one failed blind date attempt before Glenn. Yes, even blind dates sometimes require a dress rehearsal. So, by the time round two rolled around, my enthusiasm was... low. I was reluctant, at best.

She told me his name: Glenn. Glenn the geologist.

I'd never met a Glenn, and I'd definitely never met a geologist. My curiosity kicked in. Was this going to be some rugged, outdoorsy scientist who spent his days unearthing fossils and looking unintentionally attractive in dusty field gear? Or would it be a nerdy guy who hoarded driveway gravel and spoke passionately about rock formations?

Either way, I had to know. I mean, how often do you get the chance to go on a date with someone whose literal job involves rocks?

I decided to wear my long, black linen dress from Ann Taylor paired with my Steve Madden platform slides. This was peak late-90s sophistication, and I was feeling confident.

Glenn and Julie were already at the bar when I arrived, and I have to say, I was pleasantly surprised. Glenn had a warm smile and a genuinely handsome face, so I thought to myself, *Okay, universe, let's do this blind date thing!* I sat down, Julie made the introductions, and then she took off. Smart woman. She knew her work was done.

We had a good time together. Drinks flowed, dinner was edible, and the conversation was surprisingly effortless. When we said goodbye, I genuinely hoped we both meant it when we agreed to "do this again." And we did.

We dated for almost three years before getting married on June 8, 2002. Those three years were mostly blissful, though we did have one relatively brief breakup. Looking back, we both probably sensed this could be *the* relationship, and that level of certainty can be terrifying. Glenn developed a serious case of cold feet, which I now understand, but back then, my patience was thin, and my logic was, *If he isn't ready, we should date other people.*

Long story short, less than a year later, we found ourselves walking down the aisle at the Catamaran Resort on Mission Bay in San Diego, surrounded by over 100 of our family and closest friends. Best. Day. Ever. I loved every single minute of our wedding, from the ceremony to the last dance. The DJ was scheduled until midnight, but Glenn's boss paid him to keep the party going until 1 AM, and it felt like we danced all night long.

We followed the traditional script perfectly. Marriage, check. Buy a townhome, check. Get a dog, Tanner, our wise golden retriever, check. Get pregnant, check. Everything was unfolding exactly as planned.

Flash forward to me standing at La Jolla Shores the day before Luke was born, watching the waves crash and feeling like we kind of had life figured out. Soon after that day, "typical" would fly right out the window and never look back.

Some say that the divorce rate for parents raising kids with special needs is higher than the already-high national average, but the research is complex and has conflicting statistics. Personally, I don't know if it's actually higher than average or not, but I do know this: there is a lot of additional stress in raising a child with a disability. There are so many unknowns, health concerns, and appointments. And there's caregiving. In our case, lifelong caregiving.

And let me tell you what that meant to me when all the clinical language and feel-good platitudes were stripped away.

It meant lying awake at 2 AM, not because my baby was teething but because I was mentally calculating how much his specialized equipment would cost and whether insurance would cover even half of it. It meant having the same argument with Glenn about therapy schedules for the third time that week because we were both exhausted and neither of us had a solution that didn't involve someone sacrificing something important.

It meant one of us eventually became the "appointment parent"— the one who knew every doctor's name, every medication dosage, every insurance authorization number by heart, while the other one felt simultaneously grateful and guilty for not carrying that mental load.

It meant date nights were planned, and will always be planned, around respite care availability, and the unknowns are relentless. Will he ever live independently? What happens when we're too old to lift him? Who will love him when we're gone? These aren't the typical parenting worries about college choices or career paths most parents face. These are existential questions that kept me up at night and followed me into every major life decision.

Caregiving doesn't have an expiration date. Eventually, friends' kids were learning to drive, going to prom, and moving out to go to college. I knew Luke would still need help with basic daily tasks at 25. At 35. At 45. This isn't just parenting. It felt like I signed up for a lifetime of physical, emotional, and financial responsibility that most people can't even fathom.

And through all of this, I was supposed to maintain a marriage? I was supposed to remember why I fell in love with Glenn when we were both running on empty and having conversations that revolve around diapers and insurance denials?

This is the raw truth they don't put in the pamphlets in doctors' offices. This is why I believe those divorce statistics, whatever they are, exist in the first place.

Twenty-Three Years and Still Going Strong— Our Respite Care Lifeline

Twenty-three years later, Glenn and I are still going strong, though some days I might say we're just going, period. But hey, we're moving forward, and that's what counts.

Let's talk about respite, shall we? It's been an absolute lifesaver for us. Since our family isn't here in the San Diego area, we've always taken full advantage of every respite hour that comes our way.

Back in 2010, we met Kerry, who started as an aide in Luke's class at school before adding "Luke's respite provider" to her resume. She is also a cherished family friend. Kerry has been our Saturday date night hero, swooping in once or twice a month so Glenn and I can remember what it's like to have an uninterrupted conversation. She also provides after-school care at least once a week and handles the occasional weekend when we need to recharge our batteries or just remember what relaxing actually feels like.

More recently, we added Maria to our dream team. We met her when she was working as an instructional aide at our high school and eventually became Luke's aide there, too. I'll admit I have a bit of a habit of recruiting great aides to work with Luke outside of school. What can I say? When you find gold, you don't let it slip through your fingers! I like to think of it as strategic talent acquisition.

Having both Kerry and Maria in our corner has been transformative. They're not just caregivers. They're extended family members who truly understand Luke and what makes him tick. Plus, they've given Glenn and me the precious gift of knowing we can step away occasionally without worry.

Respite care isn't just about getting a break. It's about maintaining your sanity, your relationship, and your sense of self. And sometimes, it's about remembering that you're more than just a caregiver. You're still a person with your own needs, dreams, and an inexplicable desire to eat a meal while it's still hot.

Our marriage has had its share of bumps, and we've weathered some genuinely difficult storms together, but at the end of the day, Glenn is someone I can always count on to help, to listen and to laugh at life's absurdities with me. Steady, loyal, and someone who doesn't just say he's in it for the long haul—he lives it. He's a hands-on dad to both our boys, just in very different ways depending on what each of them needs.

One of my favorite Glenn stories comes from when Luke was in 6th grade. Glenn offered to drop Luke off at school one day and decided to park up the hill from the school to avoid that dreaded drop-off line. Before they left the house, I repeatedly told him, "Don't put Luke's shoes on until after you park. He gets excited when we arrive and often kicks them off. You'll just have to put them back on."

Did he listen? No. Did Luke kick off his shoes as soon as they parked? Yes. Did Luke kick one of his shoes out of the car, and did it land in a gutter? Also yes.

Being the handy guy he is, Glenn grabbed some tool out of the truck to try to reach the shoe. He must have spent a good amount of time wrestling with it because Luke's aide, Kerry, came looking for him. By the time she arrived, Glenn was drenched in sweat, but still without a shoe.

So, she walked Luke into the classroom with one shoe, only to be surprised when Glenn finally retrieved the other, soaking wet, from the gutter and brought it in.

Needless to say, I resumed my duty of driving Luke to school the next morning.

Glenn and I laugh about that story often. We also laugh about the time he took Luke to physical therapy, and I later received an email from the therapist telling me how Luke had walked in with his shoes on the wrong feet. They got a kick out of it.

These stories aren't about mistakes or frustration; they're about the unpredictable, messy, hilarious moments that come with parenting Luke.

Here's the thing about having a child with very high-level caregiving needs: it's ridiculously easy to slip into what I call "keeping score" mode. You know the drill; I wake him up at 6 AM almost every morning, I make the meals, schedule ALL the appointments, buy the groceries, remember which therapist we're seeing on Tuesday, and keep track of medication refills. The mental load is real, and sometimes it feels like I'm running a small corporation dedicated entirely to Luke's well-being.

But then, I have to give myself a reality check. Glenn isn't sitting around binge-watching sports or eating bonbons all day, though some days he probably wishes he could. He's working hard to provide for our family, dealing with his own work stress, and somehow still managing to be present when we need him most.

And here's what really matters: Glenn always steps in to handle any late-night issues or to take Luke on yet another bike ride around the neighborhood. Even when he's exhausted, even when he's had his own long day, he is present (or at least mostly present, and that's good enough). He's a fully engaged dad, making those bike rides an adventure and creating memories of his own.

The truth is, we fill different but equally important roles in our family. Instead of keeping a running tally of who's doing what—though, let's be honest, I still occasionally catch myself doing this—I try to step back and appreciate that we're both working incredibly hard and always have our family's best interest in mind. Glenn may not be the one coordinating Luke's daily schedule, but he's the kind of father who drops everything without hesitation when adventure or late-night duty calls. All-day expeditions to the Safari Park? Glenn embraces those moments wholeheartedly. And he hardly ever mutters a single complaint about rearranging his work commitments at the last minute, not even when it's the third time that week his carefully planned schedule gets turned upside down.

This willingness to prioritize family over everything else showcases Glenn's character as both an exceptional father and devoted husband. He understands that childhood is fleeting and that these unplanned adventures often become the most treasured memories. His flexibility and genuine enthusiasm for spending quality time with both boys demonstrate the kind of selfless love that defines truly great parents. Glenn doesn't just make time for his family. He makes us his priority, proving that being present and engaged matters far more than any meeting or deadline ever could.

That's the stuff that really counts. I try to remind myself of that when the exhaustion hits like a brick wall, when I've been going for 16 straight hours, running on fumes, and I'm literally falling asleep while folding laundry. My eyes burn, my body aches, and all I want is five minutes of peace that doesn't involve someone needing something from me.

But some days, it's just *hard*. Hard to keep up the level of caregiving that's expected, not just physically but emotionally. It's hard to stay patient. It's hard to be kind when every nerve in my body feels frayed. Some days, I lose it. I'm short with Glenn. I snap. I nitpick. I keep score over who did what—like somehow that's going to make it feel more fair. And then comes the regret.

The regret is the worst part. It creeps in after the dust settles, after the sigh, after the apology. That guilt of knowing I didn't show up the way I wanted to. That voice in my head whispering, *You could've handled that better*. And I know I could have. But in the moment? I was just... empty.

Love Lesson from a Mom

What matters is that you get up the next day and try again. Because that's what we do. Not because it's easy—far from it. But because it matters. Because love, real love, isn't just the highlight reel. It's not just date nights and laughing at the same dumb movie for the hundredth time. It's the arguments, the silent treatments, the messy, unfiltered moments that no one posts about.

Keep showing up for your people, the ones who show up for you, even when you're not at your best. The ones who know exactly how you take your coffee and exactly how you fall apart. The people who walk through this life with you, not just during the good and the shiny moments but the bad, the boring, and the completely dysfunctional.

Don't strive for perfection. Every hug, every word of encouragement, every moment you simply show up is proof that you are enough

Some days, you may be a well-oiled machine. Other days, it may feel like you are being held together by duct tape. But you keep going. Through the chaos, in the quiet and the in-between.

And honestly, that's what makes it real. That's what makes it worth it.

eleven

The Art of Conserving Luke (And Our Sanity)

GLENN AND I WERE COMPLETELY ON THE same page that Luke would need to be conserved when he turned 18. We weren't dragging our feet. We weren't in denial. We knew the stakes. It's a huge deal, especially when it comes to medical care. Once your child turns 18, the system just flips a switch. One day, you're Mom. The next day, you're "unauthorized." Doctors' offices, insurance companies, some school administrators—suddenly, no one will talk to you, even when your child has significant special needs and still lives under your roof and depends on you for literally everything.

I knew this. I was on it. Or at least, I thought I was.

What I didn't realize, what no one really tells you until you're knee-deep in it, is how long the whole process takes.

First, you have to find an attorney who works with conservatorships and has availability, which isn't always easy. Then, you wait for a consultation. Then, there's paperwork. Meetings. Declarations. More paperwork. Filing dates. Court schedules. Letters from doctors. More paperwork. It's a very slow-moving bureaucratic process, where the only way out is legal guardianship.

And it takes months.

By the time I realized how far behind we were, I was already playing catch-up with a ticking clock and a kid about to legally become a man.

The morning of our conservatorship hearing, I was nervous.

I wasn't expecting to feel that way. We had already gotten through what I thought was the hard part: the paperwork, the interviews, the tedious, never-ending list of legal steps. That part was done.

The hearing was virtual, so the three of us—Glenn, Luke, and I—sat together in my home office, waiting for it to start. Luke's presence was mandatory. The judge had to see him to make the final determination, to decide whether or not he should be legally conserved.

We were fine with that. Happy, even. Luke was part of the process.

There were several cases scheduled that morning, and thankfully, ours was near the beginning because there was no way Luke was going to sit still in that chair for hours, even with his noise-canceling headphones and his iPad. We were armed with our tools of survival and a tiny bit of hope that the system would show up with compassion.

There are seven legal powers someone can be conserved for in California, seven critical areas of decision-making. We were asking for all seven. Luke had just turned 18 the week before. We were only a week late, and Glenn and I were asking the court to allow us to continue making decisions for him, such as where he lives, his education, medical care, social life, relationships, and more.

As the hearing progressed, my nerves got worse. Not sharp and panicky, but more like a slow tightening in my chest. A heaviness. The kind that creeps in when you're trying to be composed but something much deeper is stirring.

We knew this was the right thing to do. There was no doubt. But knowing didn't make it any easier.

Then, the judge asked a question I wasn't ready for.

"Do you want to take away Luke's right to vote?"

In California, being conserved doesn't automatically mean you lose the right to vote. In order to strip that right, the court must determine that the individual cannot express a desire to vote, even with accommodations. The judge explained this carefully. Clearly. Emphatically.

This is no small thing. Taking away someone's voice, their say in who governs them, who makes laws about their healthcare, their education, their existence, is a huge deal.

And then, it hit me.

All of it.

I tried to bite my tongue the same way I had years ago when Luke was wheeled off in that red wagon on his first day of school. After all, I mostly held it together then.

But I couldn't this time.

I was crying. Hard. Ugly crying. The kind that hits from the inside out, where the grief doesn't even fully make sense yet. It just erupts.

Because all of a sudden, none of it made sense.

I've spent Luke's whole life fighting for inclusion. Demanding it. Advocating for him to be seen and treated like any other kid. I've told every teacher, therapist, aide, and stranger who crossed his path to presume competence. To assume he understands, even if they're not sure. Even if he can't say, "I get it," out loud.

Because he does.

And yet there I was, sitting in front of a judge, asking to take away his right to vote.

The words wouldn't stop in my head.

I'm sorry, Luke. I'm so, so sorry.

I felt like I was betraying the very foundation I'd spent years building. The tears weren't just about voting. They were about the tension that lives in every parent's heart when raising a child with disabilities—the push for independence and dignity versus the need for protection and safety. It's a line we walk every single day, and sometimes, that line cuts deep.

Turning 21—Vegas, Baby

Luke turned 21 on August 23rd, 2025. Twenty-one! Technically, he's been an adult for three years now (thank you, legal system), but this is *the* birthday. The big one. The one we've been joking about since he was a baby. The one that's been circled in permanent marker on the imaginary calendar of life.

Uncle John has been talking about taking Luke to Vegas for his 21st birthday for *years*. I'm talking table service at the fanciest place on the strip, Luke in a crushed red velvet smoking jacket, champagne popping like fireworks, and beautiful people laughing in slow motion. One of those over-the-top, hang-it-in-your-memory-forever nights.

And for years, I laughed along with the fantasy. "Sure, Vegas! Let's do it!" I'd say with a smirk.

But now that it's here?

Absolutely not.

Hell. No.

No one is taking my boy to Vegas. It was a hilarious idea for many years, but now it's just a one-way ticket to a full-blown anxiety attack (mine, not his).

Let's be real. Luke drinks *water* and *Propel*. Those are his drinks and have been forever. The kid cannot tolerate bubbles of any sort. Sparkling water? Nope. A sip of his brother's Alani? Not a chance. Martinelli's during the holidays? I offer it every year. He sniffs it like I'm trying to poison him.

He treats carbonation like it's radioactive.

So, unless there's some underground club in Vegas that serves electrolytes with a twist of lime and zero bubbles, Luke is staying home. Can you even imagine him with a glass of champagne? The sheer horror. I'd pay to see that face, just not in Vegas.

Instead, Luke will be spending his 21st birthday exactly where he should be: home, surrounded by the people who love him most.

And here's the best part: the universe, in its mysterious and wonderful way, gave us something even better than bottle service and roulette tables.

Recently, we met this amazing mother who runs a nonprofit called Sam's Posse. She donates adapted trikes to individuals with special needs. It's wild how it happened. We were riding with Luke around this business complex near our house because it's flat, and in hilly Carlsbad, flat is everything. She spotted us and invited us to see her storage unit full of these incredible trikes. Just like that. One minute, we're doing loops in a parking lot, and the next, we're talking to someone I can relate to, one of my people. No need to explain the nuances of our lives or soften the rough edges. She just got it. That quiet mutual understanding you can't fake is rare, and it's gold.

Turns out, her organization was hosting a special needs event at a rodeo on Luke's birthday. And we were going. Because this—this is Luke's Vegas.

These are the moments. These people. These organizations. They are lifelines to families like ours. They turn what could feel isolating into something inclusive, celebratory, and real.

So, yeah, there will still be a party for Luke. Right here at home. The people who've cheered him on every step of the way will be there. There'll be food. Laughter. Probably a lot of sugar. And while Luke won't be having a single drop of alcohol, I can't speak for the rest of us.

But trust me, it'll be perfect. No neon lights required.

School—The End Is in Sight, but We're Not Done Yet

As adulthood approaches, so does the end of school. I mean, eventually. If you're a parent of a child with special needs, you know school doesn't just end at 18. Or 12th grade. Or with a nice senior photo and a letterman jacket.

Nope.

There's a whole new maze to figure out. Diplomas, certificates, adult transition programs (ATPs), state requirements, IEP goals, accommodations, inclusion, independence… the list goes on.

Let's break it down. Some students get a diploma, either from the state or their school district. In California, there's even a relatively new "alternative pathway" that allows students to earn a diploma through modified coursework while still attending an adult transition program until age 22. Cool, right?

Luke isn't on that path. He's on the certificate of completion track, which acknowledges his accomplishments through his IEP and allows him to stay with the school district until he's 22.

Now, our district has an adult transition program for students after four years of high school who are not diploma-bound, but it wasn't the right fit for Luke.

The program we considered was faster-paced—great for students working on transportation training, more independent work skills, city navigation, job sites, and walking everywhere. It sounds awesome for someone else's kid.

Luke will never take public transportation alone. Ever. And I'm not going to pretend he will. We know who he is, what he needs, and that program just didn't fit.

After a couple of conversations, the IEP team and I agreed that Luke would stay at his high school. A place he knows. A place where he belongs. He's thrived there. He's supported. And best of all, he's included.

Luke's high school and adult transition teacher, Sarah, was, and still is, a gift. Inclusion is in her DNA. During her time at the school, she launched Unified Sports, opening the door for Luke to participate in unified cheer, basketball, dance, and now soccer. She also championed his growth outside the classroom, helping him identify and interview for two community internships that he still attends and where he has made friends for life.

Although Sarah was only at the high school for two years before she and her husband moved to Australia, her impact remains immeasurable. We miss her dearly, but we are grateful to still see her regularly, whether in person or over FaceTime. Most importantly, her legacy continues to benefit every student at the high school, carried on with dedication and support by the current teachers and district. Luke takes general education classes such as drama, choir, art, and ceramics, where he gets to learn, create, perform, and shine alongside his peers. He also spends time in his specialized education class, focusing on life skills, working toward his IEP goals, and receiving therapies tailored to his needs. The rest of his school day is spent in the community, where he participates in those real, meaningful internships that give him purpose, connection, and hands-on experience. One of the internships is at a retirement community, which happens to be right next to the beach (not a bad work commute). He serves as a caring companion, joining residents for activities like bingo, rock painting, and homemade soap-making (which honestly sounds better than most adult jobs I've had).

And you know what? He fits right in. He's always been a bit of an old soul, possibly a 90-year-old man in disguise, and he truly *gets* his new friends. We even stopped by over the summer to celebrate his friend's 93rd birthday.

Luke is a caregiver at heart. I think he's over being the one who always gets taken care of, and now he wants to help others. Pushing a friend in a wheelchair. Asking the residents, "You okay?" to see if they may need a little extra help.

He knows what it feels like to be supported, and he's learned how to give that support in return.

He's not just learning job skills. He's building a life. On his terms. With his people.

His second internship is at a local surf shop, and honestly, it's equally amazing.

Luke helps with all kinds of tasks: dusting shoes, sorting surfboard wax, watering the plants out front, rearranging displays inside the shop, and a whole lot more.

This place has become more than just a job site. It's a vibe.

He usually works alongside Kyle, one of the employees there, who is a genuinely good human, not to mention effortlessly cool in that "local surf shop legend" kind of way. Kyle's kind of become Luke's mentor/buddy. He includes him, guides him, and lets him be part of the rhythm of the day without making it feel clinical or "programmed." They joke, they laugh, they work, and they connect.

And here's the best part: this is how Luke learns best—when he's relaxed, included, and having fun. You can see it on his face. His body language. His energy. He's engaged, curious, and proud.

Both of these community internships are giving Luke more than just work experience. They're helping him develop real-life skills that will matter later on when he eventually (*gulp*) transitions out of our school district and into a day program, or whatever comes next.

Let's be real: that next phase is intimidating. And it's coming fast. But these two opportunities, along with his individualized program at school, have given us a glimmer of hope. Hope that Luke will have a purposeful, supported, and joyful life after school ends. Not just busy work. Not just boxes to check. Real life. With people who see his strengths and meet him where he's at.

These day programs I mentioned? I wish I had more to tell you. Honestly, I'm still in the early stages of learning about them myself.

I've toured one so far, and let's just say, it wasn't exactly encouraging.

Luke may have a 1:1 aide at school, something crucial for his success and safety, but in this program? That level of support isn't even offered. Instead, he'd be labeled a "Red Level 3" (yes, *that's a real thing*) and placed in a 3:1 ratio group—three students, one staff. Which sounds manageable until you factor in Luke's higher support and self-care needs, especially when out in the community. In this particular program, he wouldn't be able to go out into the community—ever.

Here's what really got me: Luke wasn't even present for the tour, and yet somehow, based on paperwork and systems and someone else's definitions, he was reduced to a color and a number. Red. Level. Three.

Just like that, it was decided. He won't leave this building. He'll stay inside all day. This is what we can offer. Take it or leave it. No beach walks. No community work. No flexible support. Just doors and limitations. And a ratio that doesn't fit.

I get that it's about funding. Trust me, I do. But the way this was communicated to me? Transactional and dehumanizing.

So, that's a big no for day program #1.

But just like everything else on this parenting journey, this won't be a one-and-done decision. I'll tour multiple programs, ask a thousand questions (probably more), and work closely with our independent facilitators (who speak "Life After School") to create a customized support plan for Luke. We're in that process right now, laying the groundwork so that when he officially ages out of school, his next chapter is already in motion. The good news? There are better options out there.

Our goal is to create a plan for Luke surrounded by people who truly see him—people who know his name and listen to his voice. A plan that works alongside existing programs to design a rich, fulfilling future. I have a lot to learn about this next phase, and I will. And just like always, I will share what I learn with other parents.

Because no parent should be figuring this out alone.

And folks, that's adulthood. For now.

Hormones are still flaring, and emotions ping-pong between "I love and need you so much" and "Leave me alone, Mom."

It's Luke showing us that he wants some independence one minute, then needing help tying his shoes the next. It's navigating this awkward dance between letting go, even just a little bit, and still being his person—the one he leans on when the world feels like too much.

It's facial hair showing up. I wasn't ready for that. We deal with haircuts (by me) that feel like Olympic events and a level of grooming that somehow keeps getting more...involved.

But really, this is where we are. We've settled into a rhythm that works, for now.

We've got a customized high school ATP program that fits, and a plan (in progress) for what comes next. And while nothing ever feels fully locked in, we're okay.

Lesson from a Mom

If there's one thing I've learned, it's that things just keep changing. And that's what this chapter is: growing, shifting, adjusting. Loving hard. Letting go slowly. Holding on to what matters. And showing up again and again, no matter what.

As everything keeps changing, your love has to stretch with it. What your child needs at two looks nothing like what they'll need at 20, and yet somehow your heart learns to adjust. You loosen your grip, you learn new skills, you grieve what's gone, and you celebrate what's next.

Your love learns to bend like a tree in the wind, swaying without breaking. It stretches to hold new challenges, new joys, and new fears. It finds patience you didn't know you had, courage you didn't know existed, and joy in places you never expected. And through every shift, your love grows up right alongside them, changing, too, but never fading. It becomes stronger, wiser, and more resilient—a living, breathing force that carries both you and your child through every season of life.

twelve

Running on Empty— But Still Going

Tired isn't the word. It's... something else. Something quieter. Heavier.

The exhaustion is layered. We talk about "being tired" like it's just a lack of sleep. But this kind of tired is like wearing a weighted blanket in your soul. All the time.

It's the caregiving, bathing, dressing, feeding, lifting. The appointments, the meds, the therapies. It's the vigilance, eyes on him out in public and in our own home because of his lack of safety awareness. It's managing the specialists, forms, insurance fights, and six separate portals that don't speak to each other.

Some days, it's the guilt. For feeling frustrated, for resenting the day, for not doing more. The marriage that still needs tending and Everett who still needs parenting.

And then, life throws you a curveball. For me, it was my mom getting sick. Because life doesn't stop just because your plate is full. Sometimes it just brings you a second plate.

So, how do you keep going? How do you pace yourself and stop pretending that this is a sprint when we know it's a full-out marathon? And I don't mean in the kind of "Look at you go, superhero mom" kind of way. I mean the kind of keep going that's steady, patient, and real. The kind that lets you breathe, stumble, rest, and rise again.

Let's start with the things everyone tells you to do. You know, the ones that live on inspirational Pinterest boards and in wellness checklists that make you roll your eyes—while also kind of wishing they worked.

Sleep. Yes, get more sleep. Revolutionary concept. Except, if you're a parent of a child with special needs, this advice usually makes you want to throw something. Not because it's wrong but because sometimes it's impossible.

We don't sleep well. And when we do sleep, it's the kind of hyper-alert sleep with a monitor right next to your head that means your body's in bed but your nervous system is still pacing in the hallway.

That said, get what you can. Don't make sleep another thing to obsess over or feel guilty about. And if you haven't tried the magic that is a coffee nap, do it.

Eat. Eat well, whatever that means. I don't know anyone who's eating kale and salmon every day, but if that's you, congrats. Personally, I try to avoid the 3 PM sugar crashes that make me feel like I accidentally drank a glass of wine and then did a triathlon. Hydrate, yes. Eat a vegetable once in a while. Take your vitamin D like a good adult. But if today was fueled by peanut butter on a spoon while hiding in the pantry, that counts, too.

Move Your Body. You don't have to "get your steps in" like it's a competition, but even a 10-minute walk outside or a backyard dance party does something. I'm not going to call it self-care. I'm going to call it self-preservation. And I just realized that I am way overdue for a dance party.

Take the Bath. Yes, baths are relaxing. And if you're going to attempt a bath, lock the door. I learned this the hard way. If it wasn't Luke or Everett barging in, wanting to show me the latest funny TikTok video or asking for snacks; it was Wink, our very young and very agile golden retriever, who ran at me in my bubbles at full speed, and before I knew it, was in the tub with me. Yes, my dog and me in the bath together, not relaxing. So, take the bath. Just be sure to lock the door. Light the candle. Play the music. And for at least 10 minutes, let the world handle itself. You can't pour from an empty cup, especially if your cup is full of dog hair.

What I want to share with you are the other things, the things that may not be obvious. These take time and some effort, but trust me when I say it is worth it.

Find Your Village. Some parents hit the jackpot and have family close by. Maybe you live in the same town you grew up in, and your kids have grandparents who pop over for Sunday dinners, school concerts, or just because. But when I say "family," I don't only mean the people you share a last name with. I mean friends who become family, the people who show up, love your kids, and support you like they've always been part of your life.

Now, let's be honest—having loved ones nearby isn't always stress-free. Sometimes "help" comes with unsolicited advice, side-eye about your parenting choices, or the occasional "Well, I'd do that differently" comment. But still, if you've got people nearby who love your child, take advantage of it in a way that works for you and your family.

Grandparents, aunts, uncles, cousins, second cousins twice removed, heck, even that one great-aunt who only remembers your kid's name 50% of the time but still sends a birthday card with $5 in it—they could all be part of your village. Each person plays a different role and has their own unique relationship with your child, and that's the beauty of it.

Some family members might love your child from a comfortable distance. Others will jump in without hesitation, happy to take your child to the park, run an errand together, or keep them for an afternoon so you can, I don't know... remember what silence sounds like.

The point is, let them help. Even if it's just for an hour. An hour to have lunch with your spouse, catch up with a friend, or stare at a coffee cup without anyone asking you to open a snack. You will be amazed at how much that little break can refill your patience tank.

Because here's the truth: being a better, more rested parent isn't selfish. It's necessary. And sometimes, your "village" is the only thing standing between you and a complete meltdown in the snack aisle at Target.

We've put together a local village, piece by piece, out of people who have become family. They are friends, aides at school, and a former babysitter who have walked into our lives at different points and stayed because they care. People who have seen the beautiful chaos of our family and didn't flinch. People who "get" Luke, who understand Everett, who know our rhythms, quirks, and needs without us having to give a 10-minute crash course every time we walk out the door.

And when you find people like that, you hold on to them. Tight. These are the ones who give us real respite—the kind where Glenn and I can step out of the house, breathe, and not check our phones every two minutes. The kind of respite where we know Luke is not just safe, but happy. Not just cared for, but enjoying himself.

One such person is our dear friend, Mercedes. We met her when Luke was 2 years old, and she not only helped take care of both boys, she was our friend. She had a knack for making every day feel smoother, from calming the chaotic mornings to preparing meals that always turned out perfectly. Her presence was steady, comforting, and filled our home with a sense of warmth and care.

Mercedes, Kerry, and Maria are the three constants that make up our local village. Not exactly a massive roster, but quality beats quantity every time. These three have been more than extra help; they've been lifelines. They've shown up, stayed late, celebrated milestones, and laughed with us through the mess. They've allowed us to be not just caregivers but also a couple, friends, and humans who occasionally remember what it's like to sit in a restaurant without cutting someone else's food.

Each of these relationships is special, each experience is uniquely Luke's, and each connection has made his world—and ours—so much richer.

We're fortunate to have many loving, supportive family members, and I want to share about one person who's in it for the long haul: Aunt Emily. She isn't just Luke's person now; she's planning to be his person forever. We've started making plans to travel together and to build her role into Luke's support system for the future. We joke that she needs to officially "buy into the Luke plan," but honestly, she's been all in since day one. Luke may have even influenced her decision to become a special education teacher.

Some people don't just show up for the present, but they sign up for the future, too. Emily has basically given Luke a lifetime guarantee of having someone who will always be there, always advocate for his dreams, and always be ready for the next FaceTime call. That kind of commitment isn't something you can ask for; it's something that emerges naturally when the love is real.

These are reminders that our village doesn't just lighten the load; they make it possible for me to keep going, even on the days when exhaustion feels bigger than love. They show me that Luke's world is bigger, wider and richer than just Glenn and me.

Enjoy the "Little Things." This may sound trite at first. "Enjoy the little things, for they are the big things." You've heard it a hundred times, embroidered on pillows, written in fancy fonts, maybe even taped to your mom's refrigerator. It sounds like a cliché because it is a cliché.

But clichés usually get repeated because they're true.

Still, sometimes they sting. Like when your son is belly laughing at the new Elmo video, while your neighbor is announcing that their daughter just got into UCLA. They're posting about their soon-to-be "empty nester adventures," complete with matching luggage and #wanderlust hashtags. Note to self: unfollow neighbor.

Here's the truth: as your child gets older, the gap between what they're doing and what their peers are doing only grows wider. And so does the gap between what you're doing compared to your peers. While other parents are planning gap year trips to Europe with their 18-year-olds or shopping for dorm bedding, we're still double checking his bedroom door and triple-locked window to make sure they are secure enough to keep him out of trouble overnight.

It's a different world. And if I'm not careful, that awareness alone can zap my energy for an entire day.

The reality for us is that Glenn and I do not have plans to become empty nesters. We travel modestly, but there will be limited globe-trotting around the world with Luke in tow. We're at the stage where we can squint and just barely make out the faintest light at the end of our working years. But what comes after? What does that next phase even look like?

Future planning isn't optional for families like ours—it's survival. It's part of how you keep going when you are so tired. You dream about a future that feels sustainable, and even joyful. You look at the practical things, like housing, support, and finances, but you also dare to imagine what you might look forward to. That's how you keep from collapsing under the weight of comparison, or resentment, or exhaustion.

And along the way, you treasure the little things that give you fuel. Family dinners around the table and cooking together, even when it's messy and takes twice as long. Those meals turn into treasured memories. The cuddling, even as an adult. The way Luke asks, "You ok?" 50 times a day or "Mommy home yet?" when I'm out. His innocence is disarming. Everyone is his best friend.

You learn to appreciate the mornings when you can sleep in an extra hour, the way he loves us with his whole self and feels completely safe. How his whole being lights up with love for Wink, our golden retriever, all day, every day. You treasure the trips to the beach, the annual road trips with Aunt Emily, and the ordinary days that turn into the good stuff you'll remember.

So, yes, enjoy the little things. These ordinary moments are sacred. They may not always look like Instagram-worthy milestones, but they are fuel. They're the tiny jolts of energy that keep you upright when the world tells you that you should have collapsed already.

Because when you're this tired, the little things aren't just the big things; they're the only things.

Say Yes to Self-Care. When I used to think about self-care, I pictured the spa version, with massages, mani-pedis, and maybe a cucumber water if I was feeling fancy. Looking back, that's a little naïve, like self-care was just a scented candle away. I still say yes to a good massage any day, but the truth is, most of them come from Glenn's tired hands instead of a masseuse with Enya playing in the background.

Self-care is now survival care. It's the nap I take in the middle of the afternoon when my body says, "You're done," even though the laundry mountain is screaming otherwise. It's sneaking out for a movie or brunch with a friend and pretending, for two hours, that I don't have 14 tabs open in my brain about IEP goals, medical paperwork, and what Luke is up to in his room. It's saying yes to a hot bath, a walk at the beach, or running stairs until my legs remind me that I am not, in fact, 20 years old anymore.

Some days, self-care looks noble: drinking all my water, hitting my protein goal, stretching like I'm training for something other than surviving the week. Other days, self-care is a Roche Ferrer, and yes, I meant *Ferrero Rocher*, but when you're tired enough to mix up the name of your favorite chocolate, you need more than one. Honestly, why can't I ever remember the name of that darn chocolate?

It's also knowing when to walk away, sometimes from a tense conversation with Glenn before I say something I don't mean, and sometimes from any caregiving except my own, for just a short while.

It's throwing on my headphones and blasting my playlist or losing myself in an audiobook instead of helping Everett with geometry because, let's be real, he probably gets it better without me.

Self-care is buying a new outfit for work—or at least a "new-to-me" outfit—that makes me feel slightly less like the exhausted woman who just spent two hours packing lunches while managing the bedtime routine. It's visiting my baby nephew, Henry, in Austin and remembering what it feels like to hold someone so small and uncomplicated. Or it's catching up and enjoying a good laugh with my sister, Melissa, in Minnesota for 30 minutes, so I forget how tired I am.

Mostly, it's about learning to read myself, knowing what I need in that exact moment, and giving myself permission to take it. My needs shift from year to year, month to month, and sometimes hour to hour. Some days, I need kale. Some days, I need carbs. Some days, I need silence. Some days, I need my village to scoop me up and remind me I'm not in this alone.

Self-care means prioritizing myself some of the time. Because if I burn out completely, the whole ship may go down. Glenn, Luke, Everett—everyone needs me afloat. Saying yes to self-care is really just saying yes to keeping our family and myself alive and moving forward, one tired but determined step at a time.

Love Lessons from a Mom

Love is never a solo act. It takes a village, whether that's grandparents down the street, a trusted aide who becomes family, or a sister who signs up for the long haul. Love means letting people in, even when it feels easier to do everything yourself. Because sometimes the most loving thing you can do for your child is to hand the reins, even briefly, to someone you trust.

And for single parents or those living with limited resources, your village is out there. It can be neighbors who trade babysitting for errands, school staff who get it, parents you meet at the playground, community programs, local libraries, early intervention groups, or even online networks of parents who live parallel lives.

Love is also learning to see the "little things" as the fuel that keeps you going—a laugh around the dinner table, a road trip tradition, the sound of your child calling your name. Ordinary moments become sacred when you realize they're the moments that truly matter.

And love, finally, is survival care. It's saying yes to naps, carbs, walks, chocolate, and space when you need it. It's knowing you can't give your best when you're running on empty and giving yourself permission to refill in whatever way keeps you afloat.

The truth is, this kind of love isn't always soft and sentimental. It's strong, gritty, and practical. It's the love that builds a village, treasures the ordinary, and fights to keep showing up, day after day.

Because the greatest act of love you can give your family is a version of you who is still standing, still laughing, and still able to love them back with your whole heart.

thirteen

THE LONG GAME

WHEN I SAY "THE LONG GAME," I'M not at all talking about fixing your child. There's nothing to fix. Let me repeat that for the doubters: THERE. IS. NOTHING. TO. FIX. It's not about hitting milestones on someone else's timeline or checking boxes someone else made. The long game is showing up every day, loving fiercely, being present, and keeping at it even when it's messy, exhausting, and invisible to everyone else. It's persistence over perfection. It's hope over panic. It's believing that the small, consistent acts matter more than anyone's checklist.

Our long game is made up of those small, consistent acts that have allowed Luke to flourish like a mountain stream carving its path through stone—relentless, sparkling, and utterly himself.

He is happy. Genuinely happy a lot of the time. Happy in ways that might make adults a little envious.

His speech continues to grow and expand, which in Luke's case, is sometimes therapist speak for "this kid won't shut up." He talks. A lot. Like, *A LOT,* a lot. We used to pray for words, any words. We celebrated "more" and "all done" like it was an Oscar after-party. We filmed "mommy" like we'd discovered fire. And now? Now, we're watching Luke narrate every single thing he sees, thinks, or wonders about.

In fact, we never thought we'd have to tell him to *stop* talking. We laugh with his speech and language therapist at school because the kid is absolutely, gloriously unstoppable. We reminisce, "Remember when we thought he'd never be a verbal communicator?" Yes, I remember.

Here's another tip for anyone navigating the beautiful chaos of raising a neurodivergent child: don't listen to the doctors who say, "If they don't do this by age _____, they never will." Pfft—that's me scoffing. That is misleading advice that may be accompanied by a medical degree, but that doesn't make it right.

Reality check! Kids have their own schedules. Some march to their own drum. Some create entirely new instruments. Some just start dancing when the world isn't looking, then moonwalk their way into milestones everyone said were impossible. Luke is living, breathing, chattering proof that timelines are suggestions, not laws.

When the World Is Not Kind

There are a lot of good people out there. Many of them will smile at your child's quirks, laugh at their jokes, and marvel at their abilities. Luke has a chromosome disorder, and unlike some other diagnoses, it is very apparent from first glance that Luke has special needs. It's a blessing and a curse. Many people are kind, but many also underestimate him right off the bat. But sometimes, the world makes its ugliness spectacularly obvious.

Recently, on a trip to see my sister, we were out walking around her neighborhood, just a normal Sunday evening getting in our steps. It had been a great day, checking out a few new sites. Luke was in his element, hanging with his person, Aunt Emily.

Then, a man walked towards us, maybe in his 30s, with earbuds in and nothing about him that would have made me take a second glance. Until he spoke.

He looked at me, looked at Luke (who was probably mid-sentence about something wonderfully random), then looked back at me like I owed him an explanation for existing. And then, with pure, venomous rage that belonged in a different century, said, *"F***ing R-word."*

I froze. Not the kind of freeze like when you're trying to remember if you locked the door. The kind of freeze that happens when someone sucker-punches your soul right there on the street. Hurt, scared, furious for Luke, who, thank goodness, was too busy being amazing to fully process what had just happened.

My brain went into overdrive. *Do I scream? Do I educate? Do I cry?* I did none of those things. What I did was look at Glenn and tell him to let it go. Let. It. Go. Our safety comes first. We do not know who this man is or why he is so full of rage, so let it go. He did. Reluctantly.

Meanwhile, my heart was breaking because we work so hard, every day, in every interaction, with every tiny step forward that we celebrate like New Year's Eve, and here comes this stranger who is so angry. Why? Maybe it's because he assumes Luke depends on government assistance, and Luke's very existence is nothing but a burden on him. Or maybe because society still doesn't understand that different doesn't mean broken. The truth is that I don't know why someone would say something so hurtful. I wanted to scream at him, "This child brings more joy to the world in one random Tuesday than you've managed in your entire miserable existence. This child is living, learning, thriving, and contributing to society in ways your small brain can't even comprehend."

But I didn't say that. Because sometimes protecting your child means you have to swallow your rage and keep moving forward.

And I refuse to give that man any more of my headspace.

That moment is exactly why I help organize assemblies at school. That's why I speak up at IEP meetings and make everyone slightly uncomfortable when I talk about inclusion. That's why I try to spread the word to end the "R-word," even when some people roll their eyes and say, "It's just a word."

Just a word. Right. Just like "love" is just a word. Just like "hope" is just a word.

Sometimes it feels like you're screaming into the void. Sometimes you wonder if any of this advocacy matters. Sometimes you lie awake at night wondering if you're doing enough, being enough, fighting hard enough for your kid.

But then, Luke laughs—this pure, infectious sound that makes strangers smile from across parking lots. Or he says something so clever that you have to write it down because no one would believe it. Or he hugs you out of nowhere, just because, and suddenly the world makes sense again.

And I remember that the long game isn't about immediate change. Sometimes change happens so slowly you don't even notice it. It's not about visible progress; it's about persistence. It's about showing up every single day, even when the world tries to tell you that your child's existence is somehow inconvenient.

It's about teaching Luke and others that he belongs here, that his voice matters, that his way of seeing the world isn't something to apologize for. It's about teaching the world that different is not less, that milestones come in all shapes and sizes, and that joy doesn't fit neatly into boxes.

We keep going because hope isn't optional; it's the fuel that keeps the whole machine running. Love isn't optional; it's the foundation everything else is built on. Presence isn't optional; it's the gift we give our children every day when we show up with messy hair, coffee breath, and all the rest. Persistence isn't optional; it's the champagne moments when all the hard work pays off: first words, first steps, first time eating in a restaurant, first flight, first friend, first whatever you have been working for. And advocacy isn't optional; sometimes it's the middle finger we raise to every person who underestimates our kids.

Eventually, little by little, the world will see Luke for who he really is: joy wrapped in human form, a person with thoughts and dreams and terrible jokes, a force of nature who makes everything better just by being himself.

Mostly, yes, it's beautiful. The kind of beauty that changes you from the inside out, that makes you understand what unconditional love means, that teaches you to see the world through eyes that notice everything and judge nothing.

The long game? It's not about fixing anything. It's about protecting, nurturing, and celebrating everything that was never broken in the first place.

Love Lesson from a Mom

Love is refusing to let anyone's cruelty define any part of your child's story. It's remembering that your child's laughter, their joy, their very existence speaks louder than any hateful word ever could.

It's choosing to protect their sense of worth, even when the world whispers otherwise, and to celebrate the moments that prove their light cannot be dimmed.

Because the long game isn't about silencing the ugliness. It's about refusing to carry it with you, instead holding onto the love, joy, and resilience that will shape their life far more than any moment of cruelty ever could.

conclusion

A Letter to My Former Self—and to Anyone Else Who Needs It

Hey, brand new mom. Special needs mom. Brand new special needs mom. Welcome to a club you never thought you'd join, but here you are.

It's me, you, 20 years from now. I'm writing this from the kitchen table where I'm currently watching our son, yes, OUR son, the one you're terrified about right now, eating his favorite food (a banana) and playing with Wink (his best, furry friend). He's 20 now, and spoiler alert, he's a smart, strong, kind, funny, compassionate young man, and you are a proud mom.

But let's back up, because I know where you are right now. You're sitting in the car outside one of the many doctors' offices, ugly-crying into a travel pack of tissues, wondering what the hell just happened to your life. Or maybe you're at home, surrounded by printouts from the internet (stop the searching, seriously), and all you want to do is scream.

First things first: breathe. I know everyone keeps telling you that, and I know you want to punch them in their well-meaning faces, but actually breathe. The world is not ending. Your dreams for your child are not dead, but they are very different from what you planned.

Here's what I want to tell you and what I wish someone had told me back then:

You're Going to Become a Warrior (Whether You Want to or Not)

Remember how you used to avoid confrontation? How you'd rather eat glass than disagree with a teacher? Yeah, that version of you is about to get a crash course in advocacy that would make any lawyer proud.

You're going to learn words like "IEP" and "FAPE" and "LRE"—and no, they're not some weird government conspiracy, though sometimes it feels that way. You're going to sit in meetings where people discuss your child like he's a math problem to be solved, and you're going to find your voice in ways that surprise everyone, including yourself.

You'll discover that "mama bear" isn't just a cute saying; it's a legitimate psychological state that involves very specific skills, such as...

Interpreting test scores like you have a PhD in psychology.

Knowing more about special education law than most school administrators.

The ability to smile sweetly in an IEP meeting while saying, "I think we need to reconvene with the district representative present."

Translating medical jargon for relatives who ask, "What does that mean?"

You'll stumble, you'll get tired, but you'll keep showing up. That's how warriors are made—one small act of persistence at a time.

The Milestones Thing? Total Crap.

Right now, I know you're obsessing over developmental charts, marking calendars, comparing your kid to every other child at the playground. Stop. Just stop.

Those milestone charts were created by people who clearly never met our son. He's going to do things on his own timeline and in his own way. He will have to work harder, so much harder, than most, and so will you. So, buckle up, because you've got this.

He's going to talk much later than you expected, but when he starts talking, he is going to say things that make adults do double-takes. Yes, he will learn to read differently, but he will memorize hundreds and hundreds of words that he will understand and use appropriately, or at least, mostly appropriately. He will end up reading the words along with you, enjoying some of the same books you are reading together now—and many new ones.

The kid who "couldn't" do things on schedule is going to surprise you so many times that you'll start expecting the impossible. And sometimes, you'll get it.

You're Going to Laugh More than You Cry, Eventually

I know right now it feels like you're drowning in worry and information and well-meaning people who keep saying things like, "Everything happens for a reason." (Pro tip: it's totally okay to fantasize about throat-punching these people. Just don't actually do it.) You're falling apart at night, most nights, in the dark by yourself.

But our son? He's smart. He has exceeded everyone's expectations. Even yours. And he's funny. Like, genuinely hilarious. Not "cute because he's special" funny, but witty in ways that catch you off-guard. He's going to make observations about the world that are so spot-on you'll want to write them down. He's going to develop timing that would make comedians jealous. Best of all, he's a happy young man. I will say it again. He's happy. And so are you. Life is not perfect, but it is pretty dang good!

Other Parents Are Going to Be Weird, and That's Their Problem

Some parents are going to act like your child's differences are contagious. They're going to pull their kids away, make awkward excuses, or worse, treat your son like he's invisible while talking to you like he's not standing right there.

Here's what I learned: their discomfort is not your problem. Repeat that, every day, because you are not responsible for educating every ignorant person you meet. Sometimes the best response is to just keep living your life, letting your amazing kid be his amazing self, and trusting that the right people will see what you see.

The parents worth knowing? They'll figure it out. Their kids will become the ones who naturally include our son, who laugh at his jokes, who don't see "different." They just see their friend.

School Is Going to Be Hard, but You'll Advocate Where It Matters Most

Oh, Vicki, the school meetings. *THE MEETINGS.* You will sit through more of them than a corporate middle manager, only with way more at stake. You will quickly learn that "we don't usually do that" translates to "we are not going to do that," and "it's not in the budget" is code for "still not going to do that." You will hear those phrases so many times they'll be etched in your mind forever, like the worst mantra you never asked for.

But you will also find your voice. At first, you'll nod politely, unsure if you're even allowed to push back. But slowly, meeting by meeting, you'll grow steadier, stronger. You'll walk in with binders and data, yes, but more importantly, with a love that refuses to back down. That love will fuel the questions, the persistence, the middle-of-the-night emails. And it will matter.

You will meet teachers who change everything, teachers who see Luke's potential before you do, who champion him when you're not in the room, who call you with good news just because they know you need to hear it. You will meet aides who care for Luke's safety, progress, and well-being as if he were their own. You will meet therapists who blend science with heart and end up teaching you, too.

These people, hold on to them. They are gold. They will remind you, in the moments you feel outnumbered, that you are not doing this alone. They will remind you that Luke's future is not only possible, but bright.

You're Going to Worry

You're going to worry. A lot. About everything.

You'll worry about Luke's first day of school, his last day of school, and every single day in between. You'll worry about whether he's making friends, whether the other kids are kind, whether his teachers will underestimate him, and if they will see *him* or just see his diagnosis.

You'll lie awake, calculating: *Will he talk? Will he stay healthy? Will he find meaningful work someday? Will someone love him the way I do when I'm gone?*

The worry never goes away, but it transforms. It stops being this sharp, breathless panic and becomes something more like vigilant love. You'll learn the difference between productive worry, the kind that helps you prepare and advocate, and the spiral kind that is currently stealing your sleep and your joy.

You'll discover that most of your 3 AM catastrophic scenarios never happen. The ones that do? They will be hard, but you will handle them with a strength you didn't know you had.

Luke is going to surprise you. Not by becoming "more typical" but by becoming more authentically himself than you ever imagined possible. Your job isn't to worry him into a different life. Your job is to love him into his own.

Your Marriage Will Need Occasional CPR & That's Ok

Nobody really prepares you for this part, but special needs parenting can put your relationship through the wringer. You and Glenn will have ups and downs, disagreements over how to parent, whether that thing Luke just did was adorable or a little concerning, and strain from just the sheer mental and physical exhaustion. But you'll also learn how to bend without breaking, to laugh when you can, and to remind yourselves that you're on the same team.

You're both going to be running on empty and occasionally wondering if the other person has completely lost their mind. This is normal. This doesn't mean you're failing.

Date nights will be scarce at first, but you will eventually take time to remember why you liked each other before you became a unified front against the world. Luke deserves to see parents who still choose each other, even when everything is hard. Especially when it's hard.

You and Glenn will face some really hard things together, and they'll make your relationship stronger in the end.

You're Going to Become an Expert in Things You Never Wanted to Know

Chromosomes, muscle tone, sensory processing, executive functioning, social skills training, behavioral interventions—you're going to accidentally get a master's degree in child development just by living your life.

You'll know more about your child's brain than some of the professionals treating him. You'll become fluent in therapist-speak and comfortable advocating for services you didn't know existed until now.

And yes, you're going to have strong opinions about food dyes and screen time and the importance of routine. And then, you're going to realize that in order to stay sane, you have to live by *everything in moderation.* There will be times when it feels like the rules change every single day. Own that hypocrisy.

The Future is Brighter than You Think It Will Be

Right now, you're probably scared about independence, relationships, college, and careers. You're wondering if Luke will ever drive, live on his own, find love, or be happy.

The truth is, he won't do or have all of those things, but those were your dreams, not his. He does so many things independently. He has the best friends of all ages. He loves helping others and helping around the house. Sure, he may not drive a car, but you should see how he lights up riding his trike. He has two supported-work internships and the work is meaningful. And Vicki, he's happy.

Is his path different than you imagined? Absolutely. Is it less wonderful? It's different wonderful. Will you still spiral down the *"Will he ever"* path? Sometimes, but you'll always find your way back.

Trust Your Gut

You're going to encounter a lot of very educated professionals who know nothing about Luke or his diagnosis. Some will be amazing. Others will make you want to ask for their supervisor's phone number, and you'll make a couple of those calls. You'll even fire a few of them.

When someone tells you that Luke "can't," or "won't," or "will never" and every fiber of your being disagrees, trust that instinct. You know him better than anyone. You see potential that others miss. You understand his unique brand of logic.

That doesn't mean ignoring professional advice, but it does mean you get the final vote on what's right for him and your family.

You're Going to Be Okay

I know you feel broken right now. Like someone rewrote your story without asking permission. Like you're improvising parenthood without a script, literally.

But you're going to discover strength you didn't know you had. You're going to develop patience that would impress monks. You're going to learn to celebrate victories that other parents never even notice, and those celebrations are going to be so much sweeter because you know how hard-won they are.

You're going to raise a human being who sees the world through his own unique lens and shares that perspective with everyone lucky enough to know him. You're going to watch him develop empathy that comes from understanding what it feels like to be different and kindness that comes from people who showed him kindness when he needed it most.

And Finally...

That little boy who's worrying you so much right now? He's going to change you in ways that make you grateful this is the path you're walking. He's going to teach you things about love, acceptance, and joy that you never could have learned any other way.

The mother you're becoming—the fierce, knowledgeable, advocacy warrior version of yourself—is someone you're proud to be. The relationship you're building with Luke is going to be deeper and more authentic than anything you imagined possible. And that goes for son #2 as well (sorry for the spoiler).

So, take a break from the middle-of-the-night internet searches. Step away from the comparison trap. Stop explaining your child's existence to people who don't deserve explanations.

Remember the albino koala bear—rare, fragile, unexpected. I

didn't know then that he must also have been strong and resilient. I know that image symbolizes fear for you right now, and you are asking yourself, *How do I care for something so different, so exposed, so vulnerable to the world?*

Now, years later, I see it differently. Raising Luke has shown me that the albino koala is not a creature to pity but a creature to marvel at. He is rare, yes, but rare does not mean less. Rare means extraordinary. Rare means you stop, you notice, you care, and you learn.

The world may not always understand, and it may not always be kind. But just like that koala, Luke doesn't need the world's permission to exist. He is here, he is thriving, and he is loved beyond measure.

I know you feel like you are raising a fragile rarity, but you are also raising a wonder. And yes, it will be exhausting. Yes, it will break your heart in ways you never saw coming. But it will also fill your life with a love so fierce, so pure, that you'll never again look at the world the same way.

You will eventually learn that the albino koala was never a warning. He was a promise.

Love,
Future You

P.S. Start drinking good coffee now. You're going to need it, and life's too short for bad caffeine. Also, those parenting books gathering dust on your shelf? Donate them. They don't have a chapter on your kid. Trust me, you'll write your own manual as you go, and it'll be way better than anything published.

P.P.S. He's going to be fine. More than fine. He's going to be exactly who he's supposed to be, and you're going to be so proud to be his mom.

Acknowledgements

First, to Luke, the heart of this book and the reason I became the mother, advocate, and human I am today. Thank you for your light, your laughter, and your resilience. You have taught me more about hard work, courage, and joy than any book ever could. Everything here is because of you, and for you.

Everett, thank you for growing up beside your brother with patience and empathy. Your compassion, thoughtfulness, and independence inspire me every day. I am so proud of the kind, caring person you continue to become.

And to Glenn, thank you for standing with me through every decision, every late-night worry, and every leap of faith. Your steady belief in our family has carried me farther than you know. I love you more than words can express.

To my mom, who was Luke's fiercest champion in every way that matters. You were the first person who understood that Luke would change our world, and you believed in him—and in me—with a depth I still feel every day. As a writer yourself, I hope this book makes you proud.

Dad, thank you for modeling the value of hard work and unconditional love. Your guidance and belief in me have shaped who I am and how I care for my family every single day.

To my sisters (my lifelines) and all my family, thank you for always trusting that I was doing what was best for Luke, even when the path was unconventional or unclear. Your confidence gave me the courage to keep going, keep fighting, and keep believing. Thank you for all the good times, FaceTimes, and little gestures that showed your love for Luke. I love you all.

I am forever thankful for our local village. I am so happy that Luke has relationships with each of you. Your support, wisdom, and love have made an immeasurable difference for all of us.

To all the warrior parents of children with special needs—who laugh, cry, and sometimes share a cocktail with me along the way—you inspire me every day, and I have learned so much from you.

To all the teachers, therapists, aides, specialists, peers, and school & district staff who have walked alongside Luke: thank you for showing up for him with patience, creativity, and heart. The progress on these pages belongs just as much to you as it does to us. You gave him tools, language, connection, and dignity—and you gave our family hope.

A special shout-out to the Shine Project Foundation, my partner in providing inclusive events in our community. Thank you for creating so many fun opportunities for people of all abilities.

To all the readers, parents, caregivers, and loved ones of neurodivergent humans: this book is for you. Your perseverance, love, and advocacy make a difference every single day. I hope these pages remind you that you are not alone, that your efforts matter, and that there is possibility in every step of the journey.

And thank you to Cori, my editor, and the Aaxel Author Group for your expertise, guidance, and creativity. Your careful eye and unwavering support shaped this manuscript into a book that I am proud to share with the world.

📖Handbook Highlights

A Note About These Highlights

Parenting a neurodivergent child can feel like living inside a whirlwind, with appointments, emotions, milestones, and setbacks all swirling at once. In the middle of it, it's easy to forget what you've already learned or lose sight of the small, practical things that actually help.

That's why I pulled together these Handbook Highlights. They're not rules, and they're not a checklist to complete. Think of them as anchors—quick, practical reminders drawn from my own lived experience. Some will make you nod with relief, some may challenge you, and some you might not need until a certain season of parenting.

A note about what this is and isn't. This isn't medical or mental health advice. I'm not a doctor or therapist. This is simply what I've learned as a parent and advocate who has lived this journey for 21 years, made countless mistakes, celebrated unexpected victories, and figured out what works in the trenches of daily life. Take what feels meaningful to you and leave the rest. Every child is different, every family is different, and you know yours best.

This section is designed so you can flip to it whenever you need a boost, a reset, or a piece of encouragement you can act on right away.

Chapter 1: Emotions & Self-Care

Practical reminders for honoring your feelings while navigating the daily challenges of parenting a neurodivergent child

* Name your feelings: grief, anger, exhaustion, joy, etc.

* Expect emotional whiplash.

* Give yourself time. This is not a race.

* Life is meant to be imperfect, so allow the mess.

* Self-compassion is important, so be gentle with yourself, especially on the hard days.

* Find small anchors, good coffee, routines, or humor.

* Prioritize sleep over perfection.

* Learn to take productive naps.

Chapter 2: Perspective & Mindset

Guidance to help you maintain balance and avoid comparison or perfectionism

* Trade comparison for connection; don't compare your journey to other families.

* Seasons shift and change. Allow yourself to ebb and flow.

* Don't ever chase perfection.

* Progress isn't linear; forward and backward are both part of the journey.

* Look for the growth. It often shows up in unexpected places.

* Celebrate wins, small and large.

* Focus on your child, not the checklist.

Chapter 3: Love Lessons in Everyday Parenting

Simple, daily ways to stay emotionally connected and remind your child they are deeply seen and loved

* Prioritize one-on-one attention.

* Follow their lead.

* Check in emotionally, not just physically.

* Be consistent, not perfect.

* Celebrate small victories.

* Accept your limits. You can't do it all.

* Use touch or gestures that feel safe and comforting.

* Share your own feelings in an age-appropriate way.

* Create small rituals or routines together.

* Notice and comment on their efforts and strengths.

* Make time for playful moments every day.

* Offer choices to empower their voice.

* Be fully present, even for a few minutes.

Chapter 4: Balance and Redefining Success

Strategies for letting go of perfection and redefining what thriving looks like for your family

* Balance isn't about doing it all; it's about choosing what matters most.

* Sometimes walking away from "success" is the bravest step forward.

* Working at your child's speed isn't falling behind; it's finding joy in the small moments.

* Permission to pause is not failure; it's part of the journey.

* Reinvention rarely happens in one big leap; it happens in small, stubborn acts of saying yes to what matters.

* Learn to say "no" to some things without guilt; it creates space for what truly matters.

* Trust your instincts. They know your family better than anyone else.

Chapter 5: Parenting & Engagement

Tips for showing up, celebrating effort, and staying connected with your child

* Parenting is about showing up, especially when it's hard.

* Little moments of joy add up—a shared smile, a silly joke, or a bedtime song.

* Your love is felt, and it anchors your child.

* Growth comes from effort, not perfection.

* Joys often slips in quietly and can arrive in the smallest way.

* It's ok to grieve and love at the same time.

* Flexibility is key. Life rarely goes as planned.

Chapter 6: Safety & Environment

Practical strategies for keeping your child safe while supporting independence

✳ Teach safety; show your child how to make good choices.

✳ Encourage problem-solving. Let them think through safe options.

✳ Create safe, adaptable home spaces. Independence grows in safe spaces.

✳ Anticipate challenges with medical interventions.

✳ Prioritize your child's dignity and voice.

✳ Use visual cues or reminders to reinforce safety.

✳ Let them try. With a net, safety and growth do coexist.

Chapter 7: Advocacy & Education

Tips for navigating school systems and advocating effectively for inclusion

This section of highlights goes a step beyond Chapter 5 because advocacy is my sweet spot. I share extra practical tips and strategies here, and if you want to dive even deeper, stay tuned for my second book, packed with actionable special education advocacy guidance.

* Inclusion = belonging, not just presence.

* Advocate consistently.

* Support meaningful participation.

* Call an IEP meeting whenever needed.

* Bring a friend or advocate to your IEP meetings.

* Seek support from parent networks, advocates, or online communities. You're stronger when you're not alone.

* Familiarize yourself with IDEA, Section 504, and state-specific special ed laws. Knowledge is power at IEP meetings.

* Request written copies of all evaluations, IEPs, progress reports, and work samples a few days before the IEP meeting. You can't advocate for what you don't know, and planning is key.

* Keep a binder or digital folder with everything: assessments, notes from meetings, correspondence, and observations.

* Track progress and challenges at home and school. It helps you provide clear examples when discussing support and services.

* Document conversations; follow up verbally discussed points with a brief email summary.

* Be specific, not general. Instead of "They struggle with reading," say "They need 1:1 phonics support for decoding multi-syllable words."

* Ask open-ended questions: "Can you show me how you're measuring progress in math?"

* Collaborate with teachers and therapists as much as possible. Partners are more receptive when you show you understand their perspective.

* Attend school events or volunteer, when possible. Visibility can help staff see your child as more than a label.

* Don't wait for problems to escalate. Call IEP meetings as needed.

* Know that advocacy isn't a one-time event; it's ongoing. Small, consistent check-ins often prevent bigger conflicts later.

* Ask about assistive technology, alternative curriculum approaches, or community-based experiences if traditional methods aren't working.

Chapter 8: Therapy & Progress Tracking

Guidelines for supporting therapies, consistency, and tracking growth

* Teach dignity through respect.

* Always create safe spaces for you and your loved ones.

* Love is sometimes layered with grief and hope.

* Balance compassion with endurance.

* Communicate openly with therapists and educators for consistency.

* Reflect regularly on what strategies are working and adjust as needed.

* Celebrate effort, not just outcomes, to build confidence.

* Incorporate therapy into everyday routines for natural practice.

* Remember that love is persistence in small daily acts.

* Support therapy adherence through creativity and motivation.

* Set realistic, achievable goals and celebrate milestones.

Chapter 9: Safety and Traveling with Your Child

Tips to make travel possible— and even enjoyable

* Double-check locks, gates, and exits. Your child will surprise you the moment you let your guard down.

* Build travel routines: call TSA Cares, pre-plan seating, pack snacks, and bring comfort items (iPad, headphones, stuffed animals).

* Hotel or rental? Think "Luke-proof"—move sharp objects, pad furniture, and take photos before rearranging.

* Restaurants require strategy. Scout the table, keep items out of reach, order fast, and keep your child involved.

* Use a family "code word" (like butterfly) to silently signal when it's time to pause and prevent escalation.

* Remember: you are THAT family, and that's okay. Showing up, even imperfectly, is still showing up.

Chapter 10: Marriage and Partnership in Special Needs Parenting

How to keep your relationship steady in everyday moments

* Marriage with special needs parenting isn't just about balance; it's about constant adjusting.

* Respite care is not a luxury; it's a lifeline for your marriage, your sanity, and your identity.

* Don't keep score. Caregiving looks different for each partner, but both roles matter deeply.

* Presence and persistence are always more important than perfection.

* Extended caregivers who "get" your child can become family. Invest in these relationships.

* Arguments and exhaustion don't mean failure; they mean you're human.

* Regret will creep in, but so will repair and apology. Trying again matters more than "getting it right."

* Love is built in the in-between moments—the duct tape days more than the highlight reel.

* Keep showing up for your people, especially when it's hard. That's where real love lives.

Chapter 11: Transitioning into Adulthood

Ways to prepare for adulthood

* Start early on conservatorship (or alternatives). The process takes months, and your child legally becomes an "adult" overnight at 18.

* Know the seven legal areas of conservatorship and be prepared for hard questions (like voting rights). Expect both practical and emotional weight.

* Don't settle for "what's available" in adult transition programs. Push for placements that fit your child's needs and personality. Create what isn't available.

* Look for meaningful, community-based internships. Joy and belonging matter as much as skill-building.

* Tour day programs with a critical eye—ratios, community access, individualized support. Don't accept labels that reduce your child to a number.

* Build a future plan with trusted allies (independent facilitators, social workers, nonprofits) who know how to navigate "life after school."

* Remember, adulthood is not an arrival point; it's a moving target. Expect to pivot, grieve, and celebrate as your child grows.

Chapter 12: Caring For Yourself Along the Way

Survival Care Tips!

✳ Say yes to self-care (a.k.a. survival care).

✳ Use the nap hacks for the impossible sleeper.

✳ Eat for survival, not perfection.

✳ Move your body for self-preservation.

✳ Take the bath (lock the door).

✳ Find your village and hold on to them

✳ Let go of doing it all yourself. Accept help and share the load.

✳ Treasure the little things. Small moments often carry the deepest meaning.

✳ Prepare thoughtfully for the future while staying present today.

Chapter 13: The Long Game

How to keep persistence, presence, and joy at the center of parenting

* The long game isn't about fixing your child. It's about persistence, presence, and love over perfection.

* Celebrate growth on your child's timeline, not a doctor's chart. Milestones don't expire.

* Advocacy takes many forms: IEP tables, school assemblies, uncomfortable conversations, and sometimes refusing to let slurs slide.

* Words matter. Hurtful ones wound deeply, but words like hope and love can heal and fuel.

* Teach your child that they belong. Show up, speak up, and remind them daily that their voice matters.

* Persistence deserves champagne moments: first words, first meal out, first friendship. These are small steps worth big celebrations.

* Protect your peace. Don't give haters rent-free space in your head. Save your energy for your child's joy.

* Different is not less. Your child's way of experiencing the world is not broken.

* Give yourself some grace. Showing up with love and being present is always enough.

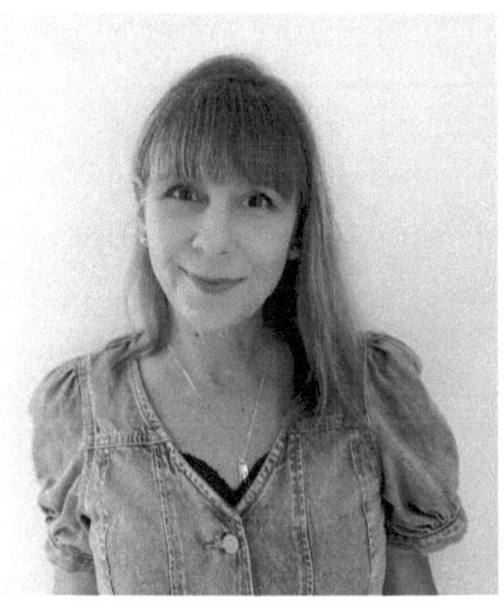

Founder of Blue Glasses Advocacy and mother of a 21-year-old with global developmental delays who proudly wears blue glasses, Vicki Christensen empowers parents with the knowledge and tools to navigate disability rights and is passionate about advocating for families through the Individualized Education Program (IEP) process.

She holds a Special Education Advocacy Certificate from the University of San Diego, is a member of the Council of Parent Attorneys & Advocates (COPAA), and co-founded the Special Education Advisory Committee in her local school district. She was also awarded the North County Consortium for Special Education-2023 Collaborative Parent Appreciation Award and organizes inclusive community events.

Vicki supports parents and guardians of students in special education by providing effective advocacy strategies to foster positive, collaborative relationships at school. Her work, both in advocacy and in parenting, combines expertise, empathy, and firsthand insight, making her uniquely qualified to guide and inspire families navigating the challenges and triumphs of raising a neurodivergent child.

Vicki resides in San Diego with her husband, 2 sons, and golden retriever where she is deeply connected to the special needs community.

Learn more at www.blueglassesadvocacy.com
or on Instagram @blueglassesadvocacy